Praise for Diane Ruth Shewmaker and ALL LOVE

I have had the distinct honor of co-teaching with Diane and experiencing firsthand the desire she has to help people on their spiritual paths. Writing a book is no easy matter. It takes dedication and a love of sharing knowledge to open gateways for people to explore on a deep spiritual level who they can be, for themselves and for others. This book is one of those tools that should be on every healer's shelf as well in the libraries of those who are just taking their first steps in understanding healing energy, and the underlying truth that when it is all written and said—it is truly—ALL LOVE.

Mary Ruth Van Landingham, SSR Master Teacher, and owner of Terra Christa Shop & Healing Center
Vienna, Virginia

Diane Shewmaker's gentle, clear energy and her professional background in therapeutic counseling, along with her thorough knowledge of the ancient energetic healing systems of Sekhem-Seichim-Reiki and SKHM, ensures that this is a remarkably clear and useful book for those wishing to learn about this powerful energy healing system and how it can be put to use.

Jane H. Hayden, owner of The Alchemists, Books and Gifts for Nurturing the Soul
Richmond, Virginia

I discovered Sekhem-Seichim-Reiki in 1997 over the course of three sessions with gifted catalyst Diane Shewmaker. The first encounter in her healing studio was an unforgettable awakening to the power of energy healing. I experienced a profound impact on all levels as the karmic roots of a long-standing health issue all at once became clear to me. A physical healing resulted.

Sekhem-Seichim-Reiki is a powerful healing technology and Diane Shewmaker is a rare kind of healer. With compassionate non-judgment she leads clients on a journey deep into the heart and its myriad wounds, where the keys to self healing lie.

Lori Lothian, Professional Clairvoyant
Annapolis, Maryland

This book is a gift for healers everywhere. It is filled with clear, practical advice beneficial in negotiating the business aspects of a healing arts practice, while honoring spirit in all that we do.

Karen L. Meengs, JD, Attorney, Author & Publisher of The Holistic & Metaphysical Resource Book
Great Falls, Virginia

ALL LOVE

A Guidebook for Healing with
Sekhem-Seichim-Reiki and SKHM

Other Books by Diane Ruth Shewmaker

ALL LOVE FOR TEACHERS: A Manual for Teaching
Sekhem-Seichim-Reiki and SKHM (forthcoming in 2000).

ALL LOVE

A Guidebook for Healing with Sekhem-Seichim-Reiki and SKHM

Diane Ruth Shewmaker

Foreword by Patrick Scott Zeigler

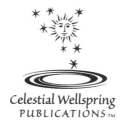

Celestial Wellspring
PUBLICATIONS™

Cover and Book Design:	Lesley Stoune
Illustrations:	Lesley Stoune, © 1999.
Back Cover Drawing:	Wendy Bush Hackney, © 1999.
Author Photo:	H & H Photo by Michael Tasto and Ann Lucabaugh, © 1999.
Logo Artwork:	Wendy Oden
Editing:	Deborah Eby
Legal Considerations:	Karen L. Meengs, Esq.
SKHM Shenu (front cover):	Computer graphics by Lesley Stoune. Channeled enhancement information provided by Patrick Zeigler, Diane Ruth Shewmaker, Lesley Stoune and Ann Lucabaugh. © 1999, Patrick Zeigler and Diane Ruth Shewmaker. All rights reserved.

The author is not a medical doctor. The information in this Guidebook is for educational and spiritual growth purposes only. It is not intended to replace or contradict any advice given to you, your clients, or students by a doctor, psychotherapist, or other licensed health care provider. The author encourages each practitioner, client and student to obtain qualified medical and psychological care as needed. Though Sekhem-Seichim-Reiki (SSR) and SKHM complement many modalities of treatment, they are not intended to be used as a substitute for medical or psychological treatment.

Certain portions of this Guidebook have been channeled through communication with various spirit guides, masters, teachers, angels, ascended light beings and the Source of ALL LOVE. As such, it is the responsibility of the reader to exercise discretion and discernment in determining the validity of this guidance for him or her.

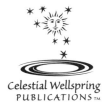

Celestial Wellspring
PUBLICATIONS™

6107 SW Murray Boulevard, PMB213
Beaverton, Oregon 97008-4467
800-966-5857 • 503-469-9292
503-469-9393 (fax)
awakener@celestialwellspring.com
www.celestialwellspring.com

ISBN 0-9674135-1-6
© 1999, Diane Ruth Shewmaker. All Rights Reserved.
Publication Date: January 1, 2000.

Acknowledgments

Very warm and special thanks and gratitude go to Patrick Zeigler, who in 1979 rediscovered and later brought to this country from Egypt the universal energy stream originally known as Seichim. I also thank Patrick for his inspiration in grounding, nurturing, growing and expanding this energy stream for individual, planetary and universal healing. This includes his genuine sincerity and active willingness to encourage the seed to grow within each person who is open and chooses to access this divine living light energy from the Source of ALL LOVE. Patrick has generously made himself fully available to me and has been very supportive of the birthing process I have been through in writing this Guidebook.

As well, I wish to thank Tom Seaman for his kindness and enthusiasm in providing historical information about the evolution of Seichim during our phone conversations, emails and when we met in person in my home. Similarly, I wish to thank Faun Parliman and Marsha Nityankari Burack for the information they each contributed and the time they spent with me going over details of the Seichim history.

My deepest appreciation also goes to my many teachers over the years who have shone their Light so that I might learn to shine mine. I extend the same to my clients and students who have provided a forum in which I could be of service while learning so much from them at the same time. I truly honor the many diverse paths of my teachers, clients and students and wish them the best life has to offer. Without these fellow companions, none of this would have been possible.

In addition, I want to express my love and gratitude to all of the members of the first SKHM training group led by Patrick Zeigler. Each person who participated in the group has in his or her own unique and special way contributed greatly to the building of our understanding of SKHM as a healing modality as well as to my personal healing process. Besides myself, those who completed the entire one-year course in alphabetical order are: Natalie Barton, Marsha Nityankari Burack, Marie Fouche and Beverly Oettle. I also extend this acknowledgment to the other group members who did not remain for the whole year. Though confidentiality precludes me from naming these people, you know who you are. Namaskar.

I extend much love, appreciation and acknowledgment to Lesley Stoune. Lesley is an inspired master artist whose tender and loving grace has contributed greatly to this work. The exquisite beauty of her heart and soul shines forth on the cover and in every page of this Guidebook. She has been by my side for this past year as an angel sent from heaven to guide, support and advise me on every conceivable aspect of making this Guidebook a reality. I also cherish the lessons of self-love we have learned from each other and am very happy to call Lesley sister and friend.

I also wish to thank Lesley's husband, C.D., for his superb professional assistance with several of the research tasks associated with the Guidebook, including the Bibliography. As well, C.D. lovingly and steadily supported both Lesley and me through the many phases of our work together, which more than once helped us to lighten up and see the humor in it all. Thank you, Lesley and C.D., for everything!

I am likewise very thankful for the many others who contributed their own perfect and special manner of assistance in helping me bring this Guidebook into form. It is wonderful to realize how many people have in some way been a part of the energy of this project. In addition to those people who made a direct contribution to some aspect of this Guidebook, this list includes significant others who I have regarded as dear friends, mentors, teachers and co-supporters, including those who have been a part of my personal healing network over the past 20 years.

In alphabetical order, they are: Frank Alper, Michelle Anderson, Eileen Bartcher, Natalie Barton, Brenda Carter Blessings, Andrea Bowman, Valerie Bowman, Dorothy Bradbury, Steve Buck, Nick Bunick, Marsha Nityankari Burack, Debra Ann White Burch, Cassandra Campbell, Stephen Comee, Deborah Cordrey, Chic Katherman, Raewyn Cooper, Kimberly Dean (in spirit), Lou deSabla, Alice DeVille, Judith Duerk, Jo Dunning, Suzanne Scurlock Durana, Linda Ebersbach, Deborah Eby, Robert Fegurgur, Marie Fouche, Andres Frame, John Gray, Wendy Bush Hackney, John and Mary Hall, Doris Harris, Jane Hayden, Shirley Holly, Nancy Huber, Sandra Kalaora, Carol Ann and Darshan Singh Khalsa, Sandra Koppe, Geri Lennon, Light and Adonea, Lori Lothian, Ann Lucabaugh, Rose Moak, Jo-Amrah Sangster McElroy, Robert McCraw, Dennis Owen McSweeny, Karen L. Meengs, Esq., Drunvalo Melchizedek, Norma Milanovich, Kathy Oddenino, Wendy Oden, Beverly and Harry Oettle, John Olsen, Ken Page, Faun Parliman, Diane Popper, Bonnie Raindrop, Susannah Redelfs, Mary Kay Reynolds, Robin Rice, Tom Rigler, Suzanne Rossin, Richard Rylander, Kent Sandman, Michael Saedlo, George Schwartz, Tom Seaman, Catherine and Allan Seller, Liliana Kilgallen Shenk, Paul Sivert, Leah Stansell, Dori Anne Steel, Joshua David and Wistancia Stone, C.D. and Lesley Stoune, Phoenix Summerfield (in spirit), Corrine Sylvia, Kathy Talbot, Michael Tasto, Mila Tecala, Susan Trout, Doreen Virtue, Ph.D., Mary Ruth Van Landingham, Marilyn Wood, Robyn Zeiger, Patrick Zeigler and Aliyah Ziondra.

My heartfelt gratitude is extended to the many guides, angels, archangels and ascended masters on the inner planes who have been steadfast in providing wise and loving encouragement, guidance and support in my endeavors. I thank the Source of ALL LOVE for life.

I wish as well to acknowledge my husband, Dennis Owen McSweeny; my son, Christopher John Olsen, and Dennis' son, Justin Padraig McSweeny and his wife Kimberly, and the many members of our families for showing me the true meaning of unconditional love and compassion and for sharing with me a place called Home.

And last but certainly not least, I wish to recognize the contribution of my pure white furry friend and companion, Ganesha the Cat, who has brought me great joy and helped me stay grounded and in touch with all that really matters in life. There was many a time during the writing of this Guidebook when he lay curled in a ball sleeping between me and the keyboard taking care to bless every keystroke.

I love and treasure you all.

Diane Ruth Shewmaker

I come from ALL LOVE

I Am ALL LOVE

I allow ALL LOVE to flow through me

I give ALL LOVE

LOVE IS ALL

Channeled Prayer from the Source
through Debra Ann White Burch - "Dreamseeker"
Sekhem-Seichim-Reiki Master Teacher
For Master David "Scotty" Haggard, 1992-1999
New Year's Day 1999

Who am I?

I am I, a Miracle.

Who are You?

You are You, a Miracle.

Who are We?

We are We,

Many Miracles, sent one to the other.

Ergo, I love I.
Ergo, I love You.
Ergo, I love We.

Channeled from Quan Yin
Chinese Goddess of Compassion and Mercy
through Diane Ruth Shewmaker
1984

Contents

List of Illustrations

SEKHEM-SEICHIM-REIKI SYMBOLS

OTHER SEICHIM SYMBOLS

A

Alpha Dedication

Come you to this place at this moment in what you call time to learn, to grow, to heal and to find and express your soul purpose. Know you have embarked on an unforgettable spiritual journey that leads to an outcome that is certain. No one who walks the well-trodden path of existing in human form is forgotten, abandoned or lost though at times it may seem to be so. For you are the true and dedicated seekers of Divine Love, Wisdom and Power. This path is one of reawakening, remembering and rediscovering who and what you really are as a multidimensional master.

Enter now into the realm of Sekhem-Seichim-Reiki and SKHM and open to and manifest the vision of your heart as Heaven on Earth. Allow yourself to move into the flow of the celestial river of Divine Love and Light and let it carry you to the sacred core deep within your inner wellspring. To you this Guidebook is dedicated. To you I am forever grateful. To you I bow with great respect, love and admiration.

Lord Sananda (Jesus the Christ)
Channeled through Diane Ruth Shewmaker

How to Use This Guidebook

Webster's Dictionary defines a guidebook as a book of information for travelers. This seems entirely in keeping with my experience of SSR and SKHM. In my work as an SSR and SKHM practitioner and teacher, I have been led to explore the vast new world opened up by this universal energy stream. Thus, one way of viewing this Guidebook is as a road map to help readers find their way within the territory known as SSR and SKHM. The information will be of special interest to practitioners and teachers of SSR and SKHM and those who desire a fuller understanding of the SKHM energy stream and its capacity to heal and transform lives.

Yet in a very real sense, all of us are healers and teachers searching for ways to restore balance to our bodies, our minds, our emotions and our souls. Accordingly, this Guidebook can also be used by anyone who is interested in learning more about the healing process, the human energy system and the application of this knowledge to first help ourselves and then to serve others. Thus, much of the information will be of value to anyone who feels a calling to heal, no matter what modality he or she may be using and regardless of whether a healer or recipient.

The Guidebook begins with the Alpha Dedication preceding this page. Definitions of certain terms used in the Guidebook are next, followed by a brief description of the illustrations on the front and back covers, an Important Note to the Reader, a Forward by Patrick Scott Zeigler and the Preface. It is recommended that the reader not overlook this introductory material as it is important to appreciating the overall context of the Guidebook.

The Guidebook is then divided into four Parts. Part One presents the basics of the human energy system. This Part lays the groundwork for those who are not familiar with the human auric field and the various subtle bodies associated with it. Part One also clarifies the terminology used in this Guidebook to describe the human energy system.

Part Two defines and discusses SSR and Seichim/SKHM, including the benefits of working with this universal energy stream and the symbolic meaning of the SKHM Shenu. This Part narrates the history of these healing modalities, recounts how Seichim/SKHM was rediscovered in modern times, and discusses the SSR family tree and related healing systems. Part Two also addresses various ways of accessing the SSR and SKHM universal energy stream, including Patrick Zeigler's approach to healing with SKHM, receiving individual formal attunements from a master teacher and directly connecting with the Source of ALL LOVE.

Part Three describes the healing and purification process, including the dynamics behind a "healing crisis." The sacred symbols of SSR are presented as well as an additional 14 symbols that are used in other Seichim healing systems. The remainder of Part Three is devoted to explaining in detail the elements of an energy session, from completing your personal preparation and getting the physical space ready, to closing the session and considering follow-up work. A section about working with animals is also included.

Part Four begins with an outline and discussion of the many fundamental qualities and values that are an essential part of being a healing practitioner and teacher. This Part then goes over important details of what is involved in establishing a healing practice and becoming a teacher of SSR and SKHM, including how to perform both in-person and long-distance SSR attunements. Part Four closes with a section describing the various elements of an SSR class.

The Guidebook concludes with an Afterword and call to action for lightworkers everywhere, as well as an Omega Benediction.

Definition of Terms

Patrick Zeigler began using "Seichim" to describe the healing energy into which he was spontaneously initiated in 1979 in Egypt. As Seichim spread to thousands of people throughout the world, other healing systems have sprouted from the original seed and use variations of the name, such as Seichem, Sekhem and SKHM.

One of these systems–the main subject of this Guidebook—is known as Sekhem-Seichim-Reiki (SSR). SSR denotes the particular system that was created by me as described in the section entitled The Sekhem-Seichim-Reiki and SKHM Story on page 11. Seichim and Reiki are both standalone healing systems that until recent years have been taught and applied separately. SSR is a unique blending of Seichim and Reiki with a third universal energy called Sekhem.

Though at times I may differentiate and refer to each related energy system separately when describing its unique historical and current usages, all of them originate from the same energy stream emanating from the Source of ALL LOVE and in truth are one and the same. Accordingly, the SKHM energy stream can be thought of as a diamond having many facets that together make up the whole.

I make the following distinctions when writing about the various healing systems that have sprouted from the Seichim seed:

- Seichim is used when I refer to Patrick's early experiences with the healing energy he introduced to the modern world.
- SKHM refers to Patrick's current approach as well as the basic energy stream from which all related healing systems have risen.
- When describing contributions and developments made by other healers such as Tom Seaman and Phoenix Summerfield and those who have followed, I use the names most frequently applied by them. This can include the terms Seichim, Seichem, Sekhem and SKHM. As of this writing, "Seichim" is the name that is most widely used and well-known.

Per Tom Seaman's request, the Guidebook refers to him as "T'om" when only his first name is used and as "Tom Seaman" when his first and last names are used together. Similarly, Marsha Burack has asked that she be referred to as "Marsha Nityankari Burack" when her entire name is used and as "Nityankari" when only one name is used.

About the Cover Illustrations

The Front Cover

The Guidebook's front cover illustration is a shenu–an Egyptian word meaning "that which encircles." The basic design of the shenu was first conceived and designed by Patrick Zeigler in 1996 and is his depiction of the infinite SKHM energy stream that he rediscovered in 1979 as part of a spontaneous initiation experience in the Great Pyramid of Egypt. With Patrick's blessing, the original design of the shenu has recently been enhanced through spiritual inspiration and a collaborative effort coordinated by me that included Patrick, Lesley Stoune and Ann Lucabaugh. Further discussion of the term shenu and its use in SSR and SKHM may be found in the section entitled The SKHM Shenu on page 9.

The Back Cover

The back cover illustration is a drawing channeled by Wendy Bush Hackney in an intuitive reading I received from her in March 1999. Wendy's drawing is a mandala that expresses the love and energy surrounding the creation of this Guidebook and my process in writing it. In addition, it is a breathing tool and a meditative focus for connecting to the in and out breath of the Source of ALL LOVE and allowing the Source to *breathe you*. Wendy described it as a moving, pulsing and radiant soul egg which carries the essence of our divinity and the fertility of the new paradigm that is being birthed on our planet today. As such, it is my feeling that this soul egg image is another sacred expression of the energy encapsulated within the SKHM Shenu.

I hope that you will find both of these images to be useful tools for your spiritual development and growth.

Important Note to the Reader

Believe nothing, O monks merely because you have been told it . . . or because it is traditional, or because you yourselves have imagined it. Do not believe what your teacher tells you merely out of respect for the teacher. But whatsoever, after due examination and analysis, you find to be conducive to the good, the benefit, the welfare of all beings—that doctrine believe and cling to, and take it as your guide.

Attributed to The Buddha, 563-483 BCE

This Guidebook contains sacred knowledge in the form of healing techniques, symbols and attunement procedures that until recently have been available only to those who have received at least one attunement from a Master Teacher of Reiki, Seichim and/or Sekhem-Seichim-Reiki (SSR). Attunements are formal sacred ceremonies conducted by such a teacher designed to open the receiver to channel the universal energy flow as both a practitioner and teacher of these healing systems. Those who have given and received such attunements have equated sacredness with the need to keep the information secret, available only to a select few.

While there may have been good reason for this secrecy in the past, a new paradigm is emerging as we approach the New Millennium: we are all universal beings equally entitled to freely access all universal light frequencies and energies without any form of restriction, judgment or limitation placed on us. We are today discovering the truth about the mystery of our being is the sacredness and divinity we all carry within us that flourishes in an awakened, compassionate heart.

The sacred knowledge found in this Guidebook can be wholly accessed only by all those who have opened their hearts to this truth or who genuinely desire and are ready to do so. Thus, the information cannot be misused because those who do not approach it with reverence, respect and devotion will find themselves engaged in an empty, fruitless mental exercise.

Once humanity joins together in unity and peace to live out the truth of its divine heritage, the healing force of the SSR and SKHM energy stream will be automatically accessible to all, and the need for formal attunements will become a thing of the past. In the meantime, the need is great for healers and teachers who can help humanity find its way through this unprecedented period of evolutionary growth and the many healing crises that are part of the process. If today you are guided or feel called to serve as an SSR practitioner and teacher, it is strongly recommended you receive the attunements from an SSR Master Teacher who has been trained and attuned as described in this Guidebook. Similarly, those who want to study the approach to healing with SKHM developed by Patrick Zeigler are encouraged to seek out a certified SKHM instructor who has completed the SKHM teacher's training class as described herein.

Foreword by Patrick Scott Zeigler

I found myself one evening in 1979 spending the night alone in the Great Pyramid of Egypt, which had been a dream of mine as early as I can remember. All my life and also in my profession as an architect, I have been fascinated with and studied the many design features and geometries of the Egyptian culture, most especially those of the pyramids.

Here I was at last. As I lay in the darkness within the granite sarcophagus in the King's Chamber, little did I realize or begin to comprehend the life-changing effects the events of that night would have on me personally, let alone on the thousands who have been positively affected by the remarkable healing energy that opened my heart and touched my soul so very powerfully.

After returning to the United States in 1983, I started to share this universal living light energy with others in classes. I learned from a spirit guide named Marat that the healing energy I was working with was known as Seichim. Over the years, many have developed healing systems that grew out of the core Seichim seed using assorted names such as SKHM, Sekhem, Seichim and Seichem. Today I use the term SKHM.

During the evolution of any system of healing there comes a time of reflecting on where it came from, what it is today and looking ahead to what it is to become. I regard this book, *ALL LOVE*, as a series of snapshots in time of the phenomenal growth process of Seichim/SKHM, beginning with my spontaneous initiation experience in the Great Pyramid and moving forward to provide an exceptional and comprehensive picture of what Seichim/SKHM and SSR are at the present time.

As in the flow of the universe there are change and growth, what is being taught and experienced today is simply a stepping stone to move closer to Source. In this regard, *ALL LOVE* presents an inspired vision of the infinite vastness of the SKHM energy stream and the possibilities that await us as we mature and advance through the transformative process of expanding our consciousness and fully integrating spirit into matter.

Throughout the years, there have been many who have contributed to the development of SKHM as a healing modality. There are countless people who have been deeply influenced by SKHM and feel an inner calling to share the energy with others who are in their lives. This has set a healing chain in motion that grows larger and stronger each time the energy is shared with another. Yet in some ways, it seems the SKHM energy stream has chosen only a few who are destined to express their souls' experience to a wider audience in the world. I feel not only has Diane chosen to write about SKHM and SSR, the energy itself has chosen her in this broader capacity.

I believe this book will serve many as a catalyst in igniting the flame of eternal Love, Wisdom and Power residing in each of our hearts. It is through this process of connecting with Spirit that we each bring through a greater understanding of the truth of our reason for being. While reading and absorbing the words of *ALL LOVE*, breathe in the energy and allow it to flow into your heart and excite your soul. It is through this process that an initiation of the heart and the sacred union of the soul and heart may occur.

Each of us who has been inspired and touched by the living light of the SKHM energy stream are part of a greater cosmic family of Love and Light. It is my heartfelt desire and hope that one day we can all realize this unity and live as One.

Patrick Scott Zeigler
Founder, SHKM Energy Healing

Preface

As we enter the New Millennium, we are ushering in a period of great change and quickening. This is a time of rebuilding and recreating ourselves, our lives and our planet. In the perfect timing of the universe, SKHM and SSR are here to awaken and assist us in growing, expanding and evolving into our true nature as multidimensional beings of Divine Love, Wisdom and Power.

The SKHM energy stream, by whatever name you call it and in whatever form conveyed, is truly a miracle and is infinite in its capacity to gently guide us through the steps and stages we need to navigate on our way home to the Source of ALL LOVE. It lovingly meets us where we are and then whispers, "You are more than that," and lights the way. There is no end to the growth possible with this energy.

I have titled this book *ALL LOVE* because this is the mantra Patrick Zeigler was given to work with as part of the teachings he received immediately following his Great Pyramid initiation into the SKHM energy stream. Love is truly the core essence and power of the universe and can be found everywhere. Repeating this mantra will open the lotus blossom of the heart, allowing you to experience greater love and compassion for others and yourself. Ultimately, this universal love will heal us so profoundly that we will come to know the Source of ALL LOVE as being ourselves. This state of unity consciousness where All is One and One is All is sometimes referred to as the Christ Consciousness and the I Am Presence.

Because it is the nature of this universal energy to express itself uniquely through each person, the picture of the SSR healing matrix and SKHM that I paint in this book may have much or very little in common with others' experiences and the Seichim/SKHM system with which they are most familiar. Whether your own experiences are similar or different, my intention is to simply pass on the benefit of my knowledge and understanding gathered during many years of learning about the healing process both professionally and in my personal life. If, in the course of reading and using this Guidebook, you are moved in a way that inspires you to stretch and expand your relationship with the Source of ALL LOVE and with All Our Relations, then I have fulfilled my purpose.

I am so very grateful to be a part of birthing SSR and SKHM on this planet and for the abundant blessings this experience has brought into my life and the lives of those I have been privileged to witness the energy stream touch. I thank you as well for being a part of this extraordinary, evolutionary growth process in whatever capacity you are serving the Light and the highest good.

Diane Ruth Shewmaker

PART ONE:
The Human Energy System

Basics of the Human Energy System

Energy is the creative life force that operates on all levels of the cosmos in many ways that are not yet fully understood. We are learning from quantum physics that all life and energy expressions are interconnected and interdependent and therefore influence everything else in the universe. Recognizing the human form as an energy system within this larger context opens the door to exploring new aspects of consciousness that are at the frontier of our current knowledge.

The following sections lay the foundation for the reader who is not familiar with the human energy system by providing introductory information about the human auric field and some of its components. Included is a basic discussion of the physical and subtle bodies, the seven primary chakras, the unified heart chakra, kundalini energy and the central light column.

Each of these interdependent aspects of the human energy system is vast and requires study and understanding beyond what is covered below. The reader is strongly encouraged to commit to a process of continued learning about these and related topics (refer to the Bibliography for suggested titles).

The Human Auric Field

The human energy system encompasses the vibration of every atom in the human body as well as several energy fields that emanate from and surround the body. These surrounding energy fields, known as "subtle bodies" or "auric fields," interpenetrate one another as well as interact with the physical body. In many models of the human energy system, the subtle bodies are divided into four main types of auric fields: the etheric, the emotional, the mental and the spiritual. For optimum health and well-being, the physical and subtle bodies must be harmonized and in alignment with each other.

The **physical body** is the instrument used by the incarnating soul while in the physical world and is the densest part of the human energy system. The **etheric body** is the energetic blueprint of the physical body and governs the level of its health. Just as the physical body has a circulatory system, the etheric body has a network of interlacing channels known in Eastern traditions as *nadis*. When the flow of vital life energy through the *nadis* becomes inhibited or blocked, imbalance or disease can develop over time in the physical body.

It is through the **emotional** or **astral body** that we feel our range of emotions and know our desires. The **mental body**, also known as the **lower mental body** or the **concrete mind**, is the home of our thoughts. The emotional and mental bodies are closely associated because when the emotional and mental bodies are balanced relative to each other, a harmony

1

is created that positively affects the entire human energy system. If the flow of emotional energy is overactive, the delicate alignment between the emotional and mental bodies is lost, resulting in the emotions running the mind. A similar imbalance will result if the mental body is overactive and cuts off the flow of a person's emotional body.

The **spiritual body** is the temple of an individual's higher self and within itself has several levels of attainment and realization as a person proceeds along his or her path of spiritual development. The **soul** or **causal level** of the spiritual body is associated with the higher mental body or abstract mind and is the place where the energetic strength of a person's pure

actions and virtues are stored. The essential qualities of the **buddhic level** are intuition and unconditional love. The **atmic level** relates to spiritual or higher will.

The final stage of realization of the spiritual body relates to full activation of a person's **light body**. The light body will be completed when his or her soul merges with the monad, i.e., the I Am Presence. This is the moment of full enlightenment and returning to one's true spiritual essence and identity. All levels of the person's being, including the physical body, become fully united in the unified heart chakra (see the section entitled The Unified Heart Chakra on page 4) and merge with the clear light of the Source of ALL LOVE.

The Chakra System

The human energy field includes seven primary energy vortices or chakras that are aligned along the spine from its base to the top of the head. The ancient Sanskrit word "chakra" literally means "wheel of light." This reflects the role of the chakras as internal generators and regulators of the life force that flows into, out of and through the human energy system. The chakras connect to the many functions of the physical body primarily through the endocrine glands and the spine, distributing energy through the nerve pathways and circulatory system which in turn nourish the organs, bones, tissues and cells.

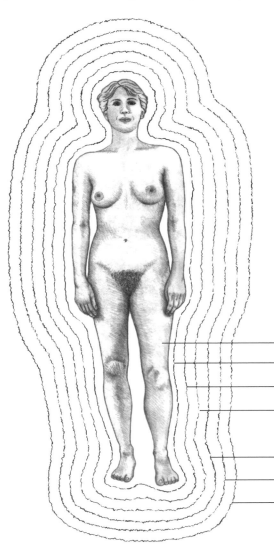

The Human Aura:

Physical Body

Etheric Body

Emotional or Astral Body

Mental or Lower Mental Body or Concrete Mind

Spiritual Body:

Soul or Causal Level of the Spiritual Body

Buddhic Level of the Spiritual Body

Atmic Level of the Spiritual Body

Light body: all of the levels of the human aura completely unify and fully activate the light body at the moment of total enlightenment.

Because the lower chakras are associated with the circumstances of Earthly life and the higher chakras with spiritual development, some cultures have placed value judgments on them. It is important to understand that there are no "good" or "bad" chakras. In Western culture in particular, development of the higher chakras has been overemphasized by many.

This flight to spirit denies the significant role of the lower chakras in creating good physical and emotional health and in grounding our bodies and our experience to the Earth plane. Just as a fulcrum centers a balance beam, the heart chakra acts as an axis point balancing both the lower chakras to ground us into the Earth and the upper chakras to connect us to the divine flow of the Source of ALL LOVE. This dynamic is depicted in many ancient symbols such as the Star of David, the infinity symbol and the Egyptian cross known as the ankh.

The chakra vortices allow for the flow of energy both into and out of the body. The energy flow from the inside to the outside of the body comes from many sources, including the Creator's life force within the person and the kundalini energy found at the base of the spine (see the section on Kundalini Energy, page 4). The opposite flow from outside to inside the body is received from other people and from the ocean of spiritual and other energies that surround us.

A less evolved person will lean toward bringing in a higher amount of energy than is given out. If a person is in a weak or depleted state, he or she will be more susceptible to drawing negative forces into the body, which will cause further imbalances. On the other hand, a more balanced individual's chakras will tend to have a higher flow out of the vortices. This attracts higher positive energies from outside the body that flow back into the person.

Each chakra is one facet of an intricate energy circulatory system within the etheric body and is paramount in its importance to our internal equilibrium and balanced state of being. Each chakra is unique, yet all chakras function together as part of the whole.

For example, if a person focuses on one chakra that is critical to his or her healing, often the other chakras move back into alignment as well. In addition, there is a vertical alignment of the chakras that takes place as light moves up and down the central light column and through each chakra (see the section on The Central Light Column, page 6). A healthy energy field occurs when all the chakras are aligned, balanced and fully functioning in an open flow.

It is critical at this time of accelerated spiritual evolution that the lower chakras work properly and be firmly grounded in the Earth, especially as the upper chakras are opened to more light. This need for a balance of the Heaven and Earth energies within us can be understood as a seesaw with the heart as the hub of our spirit core holding the upper and lower

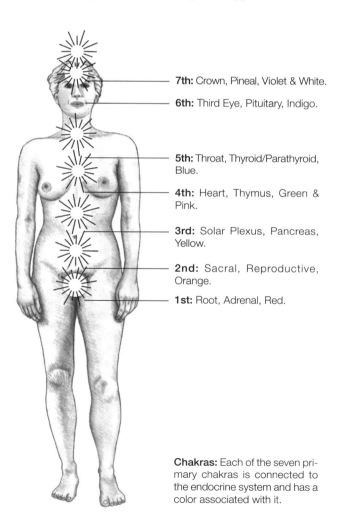

7th: Crown, Pineal, Violet & White.

6th: Third Eye, Pituitary, Indigo.

5th: Throat, Thyroid/Parathyroid, Blue.

4th: Heart, Thymus, Green & Pink.

3rd: Solar Plexus, Pancreas, Yellow.

2nd: Sacral, Reproductive, Orange.

1st: Root, Adrenal, Red.

Chakras: Each of the seven primary chakras is connected to the endocrine system and has a color associated with it.

3

chakras in alignment. This is the energetic state of equality and complete and total wholeness. When a person lives in this inner state of being, it is reflected in his or her relationships and daily life.

Many discussions of the chakra system focus on the seven primary chakras, which correspond most directly to our third dimensional experience. However, humanity is reaching the point in our evolution where many people are evolving beyond the level of these seven chakras. According to information channeled by Dorothy Bodenburg of The Tibetan Foundation and cited by Joshua David Stone, there are at least twenty-two chakras, eight of which are fourth dimensional chakras and seven of which are fifth dimensional chakras. These higher dimensional chakras descend into the former third dimensional chakras as a person evolves spiritually. Stone provides more discussion of this information in *Soul Psychology*.

Other channeled material has revealed that there are more chakras beyond the fifth dimension. Information on these higher chakras can be found in Joshua David Stone's books as noted in the Bibliography. Another model that includes fourteen chakras is discussed by Archangel Ariel as channeled by Tashira Tachi-ren (today known as Aliyah Ziondra) in *What is Lightbody?* and by Tony Stubbs in *An Ascension Handbook*. Yet another excellent text that covers this subject is *Mahatma I & II: The I AM Presence* by Brian Grattan.

The Unified Heart Chakra

My introduction to the unified heart chakra was during a workshop meditation. The leader asked us to relax by breathing deeply, then breathing light into the heart chakra while gradually expanding and enlarging the heart center like a sun to encompass all of the other chakras. With each successive expansion of the heart, we were asked to merge the emotional, mental and spiritual bodies with the physical body, creating a unified field. The next expansion encompassed the higher dimensional chakras while merging one step at a time with various aspects of the higher self and

finally, with the Source.

The purpose of the meditation is to support our transformation as we integrate higher and higher light frequencies such as those of SSR and SKHM. It teaches the physical, emotional, mental and spiritual bodies to merge and then unify. This is necessary so that the higher and already perfected aspects of a person's being can safely descend and fully live in the physical body. Over time, the entire human energy system gradually becomes attuned to the heart chakra. This allows the individual to be able to draw in a wider spectrum of love-based energies and ultimately to embody the Source of ALL LOVE without overwhelming his or her electromagnetic circuitry.

Without this merging and unification process, the lower four physical and subtle bodies will not stabilize, which can result in physical, emotional and mental imbalances. The unified heart chakra meditation also aligns the chakras so they are spinning at the optimum ratio for preventing negative energies from being attracted and attaching to a person's energy field.

During my first experience with the meditation, I felt an immediate calming, balancing and harmonizing effect and knew intuitively that this was an important tool that could benefit many. I learned that the meditation was the Invocation to the Unified Chakra and was in the book *What Is Lightbody?* by Archangel Ariel as channeled by Tashira Tachi-ren (today known as Aliyah Ziondra) as well as in *An Ascension Handbook* by Tony Stubbs.

I have found the meditation to be a powerful adjunct to SSR and SKHM and have used it extensively for personal healing, with clients and in teaching workshops. I also include the Invocation as a meditation during an SSR attunement. See Appendix I for the full text of the Invocation.

Kundalini Energy

The word "kundalini" refers to the sleeping energy or power that is found at the base of the spine in the etheric body. The kundalini energy is coiled like a serpent and while dormant, nourishes and vitalizes

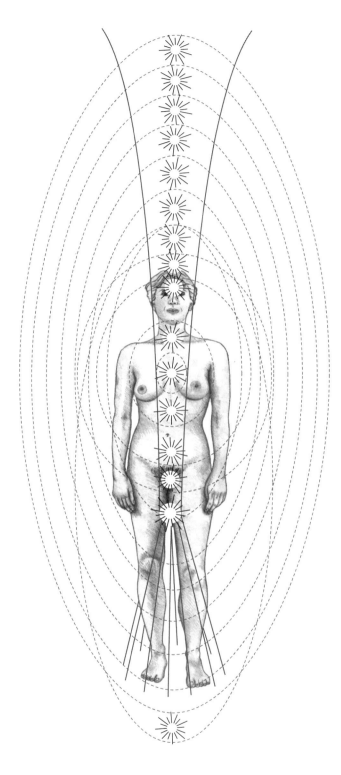

The Unified Heart Chakra: The broken lines represent the layers of intent in the ever expanding unification process. The heavier solid lines represent the grounding into the vastness of Spirit above and the parallel realities of the planetary hologram below.

the physical body. When the kundalini awakens within a person, its vibratory action gradually increases the energy flow in the chakras, clearing all that is unnecessary and coarse in the physical, emotional and mental bodies and causing a raising of the etheric body's light energy quotient. As the kundalini moves up the chakra column (called the "sushumna"), the pituitary and pineal glands are stimulated and the brow chakra, or third eye, opens revealing the subtle planes of existence.

When the third eye is opened in this way, the kundalini creates a higher visual state of existence, and the person will receive greater intuitive information from the higher realms. The right and left hemispheres of the brain come into greater synchronization, and there is an activated aliveness throughout the body and mind. It is the experience of living within a constant consciousness of the life force energy and is the sought-after awakened state of enlightenment of spiritual masters.

Activation of the kundalini does not mean that a person has achieved complete spiritual integration and liberation. It may take many years of cleansing and dedicated spiritual practice to fully awaken and safely activate the kundalini. Many exercises are available in spiritual circles and books that are designed to raise the kundalini through various forms of meditative practices and energy work. **Please note that kundalini exercises should be undertaken with extreme caution and only under the guidance of a qualified practitioner and teacher.** If the kundalini is raised artificially or prematurely, it can cause damage to the physical and subtle bodies and sometimes even death.

The kundalini energy will awaken naturally within each person at the perfect moment in his or her soul evolution, so there truly is no need to prematurely rush the process. Some signs that may indicate the kundalini is awakening include: (1) awareness of an area of physical warmth at the base of the spine; (2) a sensation of light physical pressure running along the spinal column; (3) momentary, sudden experiences of being dizzy, seeing a blinding flash of light or having a sudden surge of vitality; and (4) having contact with higher dimensions during meditation.

The Central Light Column

The rainbow bridge, or antakarana, is the central channel of light that connects the human personality and

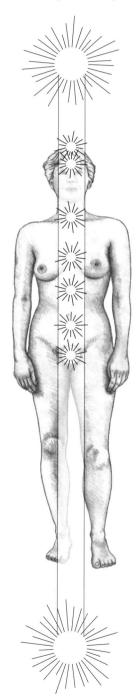

The Central Light Column: Through the integrated energy of the Central Light Column the personality and soul are connected to the I Am Presence and the center of the Earth.

soul to the monad, also known as the I Am Presence. Building this bridge of light in stages through conscious intention and meditation is essential for self-realization and soul evolution. During the first stage, the personality and the physical, etheric, emotional and mental bodies become integrated. The second stage extends the bridge from this integrated state of being to the soul. The next stage builds the bridge from the soul to the monad. The central light column is also extended through the seven primary chakras and is anchored in the center of the Earth.

The central light column is the key energy pathway that allows a person to ask for and be responsive to intuitive guidance from the soul and higher self, from higher realms such as the angelic kingdom and the ascended masters and ultimately, from the Source of ALL LOVE. The central light column also grounds a person to the Earth and allows him or her to receive guidance and healing from Earth spirits and the elemental devas, fairies and gnomes. If the column is not fully open, it will affect the amount and quality of communication between the various dimensions.

The central light column is the diameter of a human hair in a person who has not begun to develop spiritually. It naturally begins to clear and widen as a person grows in a spiritual direction. Deliberate work to build and widen the column is also necessary, however, for a person to fully integrate and ground higher levels of consciousness. Opening the column will greatly strengthen and enhance healing work with SSR and SKHM. For example, I open all healing sessions and attunements with a meditation involving the central light column. As well, a major feature of the SKHM Shenu is the central light column (see the section entitled The SKHM Shenu for more information).

Additional information and meditation exercises for working with the central light column can be found in *The Complete Ascension Manual* by Joshua David Stone, *The Rainbow Bridge* by Two Disciples and the published works of Alice Bailey.

PART TWO:
Sekhem-Seichim-Reiki and SKHM

What is Sekhem-Seichim-Reiki and What are its Benefits?

Sekhem (pronounced "Say-kem") is an Egyptian word meaning power or might. Sekhem is also the Egyptian equivalent of the Indian term *prana* and the words *chi* and *ki* as used in the Orient to denote the all-encompassing essential force that binds the universe together and is present in all life. Sekhem is both all around us and in us. Seichim (pronounced "Say-keem") is living light energy as well as an ancient Egyptian system of healing wisdom. Reiki (pronounced "Ray-key") is a Japanese word meaning universal life force. Reiki and Seichim are standalone healing systems that until recently have been taught and applied separately.

Sekhem-Seichim-Reiki (SSR) is a healing matrix that is a unique integration of these three related, yet distinct, multidimensional energies. Sekhem, Seichim and Reiki work together as a unified trinity of sacred healing energies to completely balance and harmonize a person's physical, emotional, mental and spiritual bodies. This expands the individual's capacity to carry more light and love and anchors and grounds the essential life force within his or her energy system.

SSR complements and enhances traditional medical interventions. The high-frequency, vibratory light and sound energies of SSR help to activate a person's innate healing resources to support healing of acute and chronic disease as well as anxiety, fatigue, depression, stress and other symptoms that are produced by unbalanced thoughts, feelings and emotions.

SSR encompasses the understanding that conditions and symptoms found in one level of a person's energy field usually have corresponding components in one or more of the other levels. For example, a physical symptom may have matching emotional, mental and spiritual components. As the subtle aspects of cause are addressed at these multiple levels, deeply held energetic blocks and constrictions are released, bringing the opportunity for improved health, more joy and love of living, higher levels of energy and vitality, greater creativity, increased mental clarity and focus, and improved relationships.

As the healing process advances over time, it is also common for the recipient of SSR to have the experience of a new beginning and rebirth of life together with a greater sense of meaning and purpose and an expanded awareness of self in relation to the universal whole. Other reported benefits of SSR include deep relaxation, stress reduction, clearing of addictive patterns, emotional stability and greater self-esteem. SSR

7

can also assist a person in finding his or her soul purpose, and in enhancing communication with his or her spirit guides, angels, the ascended masters and the Source of ALL LOVE. The positive effects of SSR are cumulative and will carry forward from session to session, building momentum as an individual moves through the healing process.

SSR is an energy system that encompasses the full spectrum of electromagnetic frequencies available from the Source of ALL LOVE. Each of its three components plays a specific role that when combined with the others creates a unique synergy. Reiki anchors and grounds the healing vortex of the universal life force in the physical and subtle bodies and into the Earth. Reiki also assists in the early stages of opening the doorway or portal to accessing the many levels of one's higher nature. Where Reiki leaves off in this latter function, the multidimensional living light energy of Seichim takes over. Seichim dissolves barriers to the higher self, activates and strengthens the light body and opens and enhances one's connection to his or her angelic guides, the ascended masters and the Source of ALL LOVE.

As the energies of Heaven and Earth come together to spiral, dance and become One within the heart, Sekhem balances and merges the physical and subtle bodies, unifying all polarities including masculine and feminine. The lotus blossom of the unified heart chakra bursts open and unfolds, bringing forth the eternal golden blue-white flame of what some call the indwelling Christ Consciousness and the I Am Presence. Thus, SSR is a trinity, defined by J.C. Cooper in *An Illustrated Encyclopaedia of Traditional Symbols* as a unity; a three-in-one and a one-in-three that creates unity in diversity, with the third (Sekhem) uniting the opposites (Reiki and Seichim).

At the expansive level of the Source of ALL LOVE, all that exists is fully united in the One, including each of the components of SSR. In this realm of being, there is no duality or separation from the Creator — no Heaven and Earth, masculine and feminine, dark and light, or love and fear. This is the true nature of the Sekhem energy – total oneness, harmony, peace and unification. It is this enlightened state of consciousness, health and well being in which we are seeking to live.

At this stage of humanity's evolution, most people are not clear enough to handle this high level of energy without causing major distress in the circuitry of the human energy system. For this reason, the electromagnetic frequencies of Sekhem adjust themselves by stepping down their "voltage" to meet us where we are, which for the time being includes duality consciousness. Thus, the vibrational frequencies of Reiki meet us at the foundational level of our physical or Earth existence, then flow into Seichim, which helps us open to and connect with our divine or Heavenly nature and the infinite multidimensional frequencies available from the Source of ALL LOVE.

Under the guidance of the recipient's higher self, just the right amount of pure Sekhem energy then flows into the "high octane" blend of SSR, facilitating the growth, integration, elevation and balancing of all levels of the individual's being. Another key component of this process is the building and widening of the central light column, which is a person's direct line to the Source of ALL LOVE as well as the mechanism for grounding the SSR energy stream into the cellular memory of the physical body and the Earth.

As the physical and subtle bodies of the human auric field begin to merge, a force field is created around the person that gradually allows the acceptance of greater and greater amounts of universal light frequencies without overwhelming the person's energy structure. This process in turn prepares the way for the oversoul to descend and live in the physical body. The oversoul is that already-perfected part of a person's consciousness that exists on the plane of universal love and wisdom. In this way, the SSR healing matrix assists the entire energy structure in becoming centered in and attuned to the unified heart chakra (see the section entitled The Unified Heart Chakra, page 4).

An SSR energy session may be given in person or through distance healing. The electromagnetic vibrational energy of SSR is transferred through the practitioner's hands with the hands placed on or above the physical body. The practitioner is a conduit of the SSR energy matrix, receiving and transferring it on the physical, mental, emotional and spiritual levels. The practitioner often uses one or more of the SSR symbols, which allow the energy to come forward in a focused manner and open access to the high vibratory love frequencies of SSR. These symbols are more fully discussed in the section entitled The Sekhem-Seichim-Reiki Sacred Symbols beginning on page 40.

The practitioner works in partnership with the recipient's conscious intent, higher self, angelic guides and the universal Source of ALL LOVE. The amount of energy received and integrated by the individual will be exactly that which will best serve his or her highest good at that particular moment in time. More information about SSR energy sessions is included in the section entitled Elements of an Energy Session beginning on page 61.

The SKHM Shenu

The symbology expressed in the SKHM Shenu found on the cover of this Guidebook adds to the understanding of SSR. In the Egyptian tradition, the meaning of the term shenu is the same as the word cartouche, the latter being the more modern term, according to *A Dictionary of Ancient Egypt* by Margaret Bunson.

Traditionally, a shenu or cartouche is a symbol of eternity and of endless cycles. It is a circular or oval-shaped rope of light found in Egyptian artwork that encircles and protects the names of royalty (the pharaohs), who were considered to be enlightened representatives of the gods. A shenu can be thought of as an Egyptian form of a mandala that surrounds and protects the sacred center and is the container that holds the entire cosmos and all potentialities.

Though the SKHM Shenu is represented in a two-dimensional form on paper, it is three-dimensional and is constantly moving and evolving. In it lies the celestial abode of all that is divine as well as the universal ground of all existence, which when brought together results in the perfect union of opposing energies within a person's being. Within the center of the shenu is a symbolic diagram or map of the sacred space in which the journey of the soul proceeds through the healing and enlightenment process.

The sacred space in the center of the shenu is encircled with an oval representing the cosmic egg or life principle, which is the universal symbol of all creation. In Egyptian tradition, the solar god, Ra, is said to have been hatched from the cosmic egg. The egg is the container that holds the soul's spiritual essence and the entire process of becoming a whole person. The egg is surrounded by the petals of the lotus flower, which are formed from the flow of the infinity pattern.

The soul's full potential is held in the SKHM Shenu. The shenu template lies dormant in a protective cocoon-like chamber within a person's spiritual heart center until the perfect moment of soul awakening and quickening. This heart activation opens the flow of divine light from the Source of ALL LOVE and stirs the soul blueprint of the person into motion, energizing the transformative process of developing higher consciousness and becoming self-realized. In the SKHM Shenu, the heart of the Source of ALL LOVE is within the pyramid-like octahedron structure found in the nucleus of the Sun, which is the supreme cosmic power.

The multidimensional clear light of the Source of ALL LOVE illuminates the solar disc, then flows out from the center into a starlike pattern, creating the rainbow colors of the seven cosmic rays. According to the works of Alice Bailey, these rays embody the qualities of the Source needed to bring itself into manifested expression. These qualities include power and will; love and wisdom; active intelligence; harmony and beauty; concrete science and knowledge; devotion; and ceremonial order and magic. The eighth point of the star pattern points downward and touches the tip of the center petal of the inner lotus flower, guiding the clear light of the Source as well as the rainbow rays into the top of the lotus flower, which represents the crown chakra.

The eighth point is shown as the color blue because the SKHM energy stream first revealed itself to Patrick Zeigler as this color. However, as Patrick and others have worked with the SKHM energy stream over the years, the full spectrum of colors all the way back to the clear light of the Source of ALL LOVE has become accessible.

As the clear and rainbow light shines into the lotus flower, its petals open and receive the blessings of the energy flow of the infinity pattern, which is then drawn down through the crown chakra and breathed into the spiritual heart center. This opens the stem of the lotus flower that is sitting in the vessel of the heart. The opening stem then expands into a broader column of light shining from the Source through the lotus flower or crown chakra, then into the heart.

As a person's meditative breathing continues to open the heart and the column of light (see the section entitled The Central Light Column), the column extends downward through the lower chakras, then down to the star point in the center of the spiraling Earth energy, anchoring itself in the heart of the Earth. The Earth energy then rises up through the column and meets and joins with the divine energy in the spiritual heart, bringing forth the perfect union of Heaven and Earth within the person and opening the unified heart chakra.

The pattern next emerging is that of the ankh, the Egyptian symbol of eternal life and immortality that holds the key to unlocking the mysteries and hidden wisdom of the universe. The vertical component of the

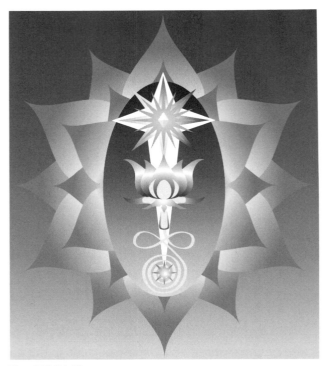

The SKHM Shenu

ankh has been formed by a portion of the column of light. As the sacred energy rises from the Earth's center through the column to the spiritual heart and becomes One with the divine Heaven energies, a horizontal flow is sent out from the heart through the shoulders, arms and hands, creating the horizontal bar of the ankh.

As meditative breathing continues to energize the process, the solar disc moves down through the column of light until it comes to rest on the center of the horizontal crossbar completing the entire ankh, which then emerges from the center of the inner lotus flower.

Thus, the energy flow within the SKHM Shenu unites the spiraling sacred Earth energy and the infinity pattern of the Heaven energy in the heart, which then brings forth the formation of the ankh. This is made possible through breathing the universal life force into the heart and allowing it to circulate and open up the heart as well as the physical, mental, emotional and spiritual levels to the SKHM energy stream. The moment of enlightenment comes when the ankh is fully formed and completely energized and unified within a person's being.

The energy of the breath is the bridge connecting spirit (Heaven) and matter (Earth) and is the essential ingredient that makes all of life possible. It is therefore no surprise that the ankh is also known as the breath of life and represents the realized human and the resurrected soul. When the gods are seen holding an ankh to the king's nose and lips in Egyptian temple reliefs, the gesture is regarded as the divine bestowing of eternal life and as an offering of the breath of life that will be required in the afterlife.

Drunvalo Melchizedek emphasizes the significance of the ankh in *The Ancient Secret of The Flower of Life* by reminding us that "(t)here is an electromagnetic energy field surrounding our bodies shaped like the ankh. The remembrance of it, according to the Egyptian point of view, is the beginning of our returning home to eternal life and true freedom, so the ankh is the primary key."

The center sepal of the inner lotus flower forms a dove, which has descended into the center of the heart from the Source of ALL LOVE. The dove is the symbol of the soul and the Holy Spirit and signifies purity, peace, innocence, compassion, gentleness and the renewal of life.

The SKHM Shenu is also the template for the entire SSR energy matrix. The spiral can be thought of as Reiki, the infinity pattern as Seichim and the ankh as Sekhem. Although they are different in their forms of expression in the world, SKHM and SSR are one and the same universal energy. Other healing systems that have developed over the years from the Seichim/SKHM seed also have the energetics of the SKHM Shenu at their core.

The SKHM Shenu can be used as a tool for healing and enhancing a person's connection to the energy stream. One way to do this is to visualize the shenu inside the heart and breathe into it for a period of time. Continue to breathe into the heart and use the above description of the energy flow as a meditation, following the flow to wherever it leads. Another suggestion is to contemplate the meaning of the various elements of the shenu while softly gazing at the image.

An individual may also tap into the vibrational and healing qualities of the shenu through toning. One suggestion is to contemplate the image while allowing whatever sounds rise up to be expressed aloud. The shenu also can be accessed by placing one or both hands on it and using the breath to draw the energies up through the arms into the heart. While meditating, a person also can hold his or her palms over the shenu while asking to receive its wisdom and guidance.

The Sekhem-Seichim-Reiki and SKHM Story

The components of the unified SSR healing system are from the same family of origin as the systems that were widely taught and applied in the ancient mystery schools and temples of Atlantis, Lemuria, Egypt, Tibet and India. These teachings later spread throughout the world, although they likely were known by other names. The knowledge and teaching of these universal healing energy streams has often gone underground at various times throughout history, only to resurface when the need for them is great. Such is the case today.

What follows is the modern historical background of SKHM and each of the components of the SSR healing matrix, including a general discussion of some of the other healing systems that have grown from the Seichim/SKHM seed. The reader may also refer to Appendices II and III which outlines the SSR and Seichim/SKHM chronology in summary form.

Late 1800's	Dr. Mikao Usui rediscovers Reiki.
1925	Dr. Usui initiates Chujiro Hayashi as a Reiki Master. Hayashi opens a Reiki clinic in Japan.
1938	Hawayo Takata is initiated as a Reiki Master by Hayashi.
1970-1980	Takata brings Reiki to the U.S. and trains 22 Reiki Masters before her death in 1980.
1979	Patrick Zeigler's Great Pyramid spontaneous initiation to the SKHM energy takes place. He also studies with Sheikh Mohammed Osman Brahani.
1984	Zeigler meets Christine Gerber who channeled Marat, a 2,500 year-old-spirit guide who was a Seichim teacher in India. Marat tells Zeigler the energy he is working with is called Seichim and gives him other information as well. Zeigler begins to practice giving attunements for Seichim.
1984	Zeigler attunes Tom Seaman to Seichim.
1985	Phoenix Summerfield completes her Seichim training with Faun Parliman and Seaman, including some symbol development work with Seaman.
1985-1987	Summerfield creates a seven-facet Seichim system, including additional symbols, and begins teaching Seichim at expos and health fairs.
1992-1993*	Summerfield begins teaching Seichim in Australia. Seichim spreads throughout the world.
1995	Shewmaker becomes a Reiki Master and receives her first Seichim attunements.
1996	Shewmaker becomes a Seichim Master. She teaches Reiki and Seichim.
1996	Zeigler is inspired to design the original SKHM Shenu.
June 1997	Following a spontaneous initiation, Shewmaker begins to channel another aspect of the SKHM energy stream, "Sekhem," and creates Sekhem-Seichim-Reiki (SSR).
August 1998	Zeigler begins the first SKHM teacher's training group. Shewmaker and Marsha Nityankari Burack are members.
Early 1999	The original SKHM Shenu is enhanced to reflect an expanded understanding of the SKHM energy stream and its related healing systems.
August 1999	The first SKHM teacher's training group is completed.

* approximate years.

Highlights from the SSR and Seichim/SKHM Chronology

Reiki

In the late 1800's, a Japanese minister and theologian named Dr. Mikao Usui was searching for the method by which Jesus healed the sick. After many years of studying and seeking out this information, Dr. Usui had a visionary mountaintop experience during which it is said that he received the Reiki energy including the Reiki sacred symbols. It is thought that Dr. Usui trained approximately 17 Reiki Masters while on pilgrimage through Japan before his death in 1930. One of these masters, Chujiro Hayashi, operated a healing clinic in Tokyo where Reiki healers worked in groups.

Mrs. Hawayo Takata was a native of the island of Kauai, Hawaii and was a small, frail woman who had come to the point of near exhaustion raising two children alone after her husband's death in 1930. She also had been diagnosed with gall bladder disease and a severe respiratory condition. Though surgery was required for the former condition, the latter one made surgery dangerous. Over the coming years, her health continued to deteriorate.

Mrs. Takata moved to Japan where her parents resided in 1935. There she was hospitalized with appendicitis and a tumor and awaited surgery for several weeks. The night before her surgery, she heard a voice say, "The operation is not necessary." Hearing the same voice again while on the operating table, she sat up and asked the surgeon if there was an alternative means for healing her health concerns. The surgeon told her about the Hayashi clinic and his sister took Mrs. Takata there that day. During her four-month stay, Mrs. Takata was completely healed in body, mind and spirit.

Mrs. Takata asked to be trained in Reiki while staying at the Hayashi clinic. Her request was initially refused because she was not Japanese. However, in 1936 she was trained in Reiki I and in 1937, received Reiki II. Mrs. Takata completed Reiki Master training in 1938, returned home to Hawaii and opened her first Reiki clinic. She later brought Reiki to the mainland United

States, Canada and Europe, teaching in an oral tradition by telling stories and through example. Note-taking was prohibited to help students increase their intuitive abilities. By the time of her death, Mrs. Takata had initiated 22 Reiki Masters.

There are many more details to the Reiki story the reader can find in the various books on Reiki. However, current research indicates that some of the previously accepted historical information about Reiki may not be entirely accurate and cannot be verified since the principals involved are no longer living. Although some details of the historical accounts may be clouded, the effects of the healing energy of Reiki continue to be documented throughout the world.

Seichim/SKHM

In researching the history of Seichim and how it came to be associated with Reiki, I came across some accounts that are not accurate or complete, according to those who were directly involved in the process. As a result, I have interviewed, confirmed and reconfirmed details with the principal players so that my narrative reflects their perspective of historical events in which they played a role.

These principals include Patrick Zeigler, who rediscovered Seichim while in Egypt on leave from the Peace Corps and brought it to the United States, as well as Tom Seaman, Faun Parliman and Marsha Nityankari Burack, who have each been important links in spreading the word about Seichim and sharing the energy. Another key principal is Phoenix Summerfield. Because she passed on in the early part of the summer of 1998, I have reconstructed her role through information provided by Patrick, T'om, Faun and Nityankari who were all in contact with Phoenix at various times during her involvement with Seichim. I have cho-

sen to write this section in great detail in an effort to clear up some of the confusion and myths that have grown up around Seichim's history.

IN THE GREAT PYRAMID

Patrick traveled to Egypt in 1979 to fulfill a childhood dream of sleeping overnight in the Great Pyramid of Giza. Patrick visited the Pyramid and found a small opening to the left of the King's Chamber created by thieves who had tried to cut through the wall surrounding the Chamber. The gate covering the opening was unlocked. Patrick did not know where it led, yet he knew this tunnel was where he would hide.

After spending some time meditating in both the King's and Queen's Chambers, Patrick left the Pyramid to prepare to come back the next day. He began fasting and returned to the Pyramid the next morning with a bag packed with what he would need for spending the night. He went directly to the tunnel and when no one was looking, started to crawl into it. The tunnel was quite narrow and tilted upward. Patrick soon found himself in a small carved-out room just above the King's Chamber where he spent the entire day peacefully meditating.

After the Pyramid emptied of tourists and was locked for the night, Patrick came out of his hiding

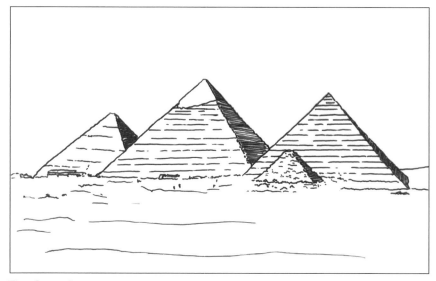

The Great Pyramid: Visible for miles, the Great Pyramid is the largest of several pyramids on the Giza Plateau in Egypt.

place and with a flashlight in hand, proceeded to the King's Chamber. He made his way to the granite sarcophagus, discovering that when he bumped its side, it resounded like a very deep gong. He stepped into the sarcophagus and lay down on the stone base.

As Patrick attempted to quiet himself, he heard a buzzing sound. Soon he recognized the buzz as mosquitos and found that his feet, arms and face were the main course. Although he had not prepared for this eventuality, he remembered packing toilet paper in his bag. He wrapped himself up for protection, recognizing the humor in appearing like a toilet paper "mummy" lying in the sarcophagus. Safe from the mosquitos, Patrick was now able to become quiet and started to meditate.

In a short while, Patrick began hearing thumping sounds that seemed to be footsteps coming up from the grand gallery. The sound kept getting closer, and he knew he had to stay where he was to avoid detection. No one turned the lights on, and Patrick soon realized this was because the sound was likely not human. This realization was so penetrating that waves of fear came over his body, almost overwhelming him. Though he had been in dangerous situations before, this fear was different and was not going away.

A presence then entered the room and the thumping sound now pulsated throughout the Chamber. As Patrick looked out into the darkness, a swirling pattern of electric blue light appeared and hovered over him. Something inside told him this was why he had come, and he went deep within his fear, reassuring himself not to be afraid.

Patrick thought, "Do what you have to do," and at that very instant, the light descended into his heart. For a moment, there was total silence, and Patrick wondered if he was still alive. Yet his heart felt so expansive, and the sound now

coming from inside of it was identical to the one that had been in the Chamber. Patrick spent the rest of the night in a state of peaceful bliss, meditating on the electric blue energy in his heart as it swirled in an infinity or figure-eight pattern.

In the morning, Patrick returned through the tunnel to his hiding place before the Pyramid opened for the day. He meditated there until he felt it was time to come out and join with a group of tourists leaving the Pyramid. Patrick noticed he was covered in a glimmering white powder and brushed off as much as he could. As he was exiting, he could hear the guards yelling at him to come back because they realized he had spent the night inside. Patrick understood their language and pretended not to hear them. As luck would have it, a bus was just pulling away. He jumped on it and it took him right to his hotel.

Once he was safely back in his room, Patrick looked at himself in the mirror, and for the first time realized the white glistening powder was blanketing him from head to toe just as if someone had dropped a large bag of flour on him. He later learned that this powder is known to be in the pyramids and is used in India to promote healing and spiritual powers. In the

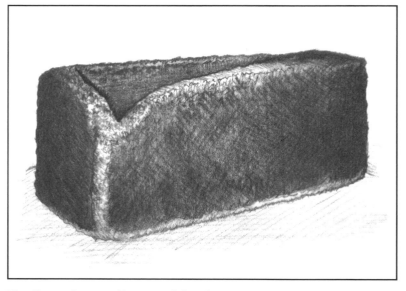

The Sarcophagus: For years it has been assumed that all the pyramids were tombs and that this granite structure, located in the King's Chamber in the Great Pyramid, was a sarcophagus. Patrick slept here!

West, some call it white gold and use it to heighten a person's spiritual vibrations.

MEETING THE SUFIS AND SHEIKH MOHAMMED OSMAN BRAHANI

Patrick cleaned up and ventured into the old city of Cairo where a Western woman approached him and asked if he could help her locate a man named Sheikh Mohammed Osman Brahani. Patrick consulted a nearby person, who said that though the Sheikh did not live locally, a group of his students had a place right across the street. Patrick and the woman found that it was a school for Sufis led by the Sheikh, who lived in the Sudan, and they spent about a week with the group.

Patrick was intrigued at how the Sufi group's practices were similar to what he had experienced while meditating in the Pyramid. Both focused on the energy of the heart. These Sufis also had a dancing form called "zikir" that was different from the well-known spiraling Sufi dance. Instead, the dancers performing zikir moved from left to right, swaying in an infinity pattern. Again, the group's practice expressed a synchronicity with Patrick's experience in the Pyramid.

At the end of their visit with the Sufis, Patrick and the woman decided to visit the Sheikh in the Sudan. The Sheikh passed along many teachings to Patrick, including giving him some prayer beads and instructing him to say "Allah" once for each bead as part of a meditative practice. This guidance came through to Patrick as "ALL LOVE," and he repeated "ALL LOVE" over and over for the rest of the week as one would repeat a mantra, feeling his heart opening more and more as he heightened his efforts.

Patrick continued working with the teachings and practices he learned during his Great Pyramid experience and from the Sufis when he returned to his Peace Corps service in Yemen. There the healing energy into which he was spontaneously initiated in the Great Pyramid began to manifest. Whenever he began to get sick, he found that placing his hands on his body would

cause it to vibrate and shake, and he would soon feel better. Within a few months, Patrick left Yemen to spend just over two years in Nepal, working with the practices and energy all the while, before returning to the United States in 1983.

BACK IN THE UNITED STATES

Though he had wonderful experiences with the energy while overseas, Patrick knew he needed to learn more about healing. He eventually settled in Santa Fe and studied massage at the New Mexico Academy of Healing Arts, which also taught energetic and vibrational healing. Patrick learned about Reiki, and during his first session, experienced the energy moving through his body as being similar to the energy he had received in Egypt. Patrick decided to enroll in a weekend Reiki I and II class taught by a woman named Marilyn Alvy. Within a year of beginning his study of Reiki, Patrick also received the Reiki Master attunements and training from Barbara Ray, who went on to develop the Radiance Technique.

As he was completing his Reiki Master (IIIa) training in March 1984, Patrick was visited by the woman he had met in Egypt who had led him to the Sufi group. She asked Patrick to travel with her back to the Sudan at the Sufi group's request. Immediately after completing his Reiki Master class, Patrick and the woman traveled to the Sudan to spend another two weeks with the group studying and dancing.

While with the group, the Sheikh's son revealed that his father had died. The group members knew the Sheikh had passed on teachings to Patrick that were rarely given out, and they wanted Patrick to become a Sheikh, marry the woman who had brought him there and teach with her. Though he was honored by their request, Patrick respectfully declined. The group members gave him their blessings and, though he chose not to become a Sheikh, encouraged Patrick to teach what he had learned from their leader. Patrick returned home and moved to California that summer.

MARAT

From the beginning, Patrick has considered the development and understanding of Seichim to be a collaborative effort. Shortly after arriving in California, Patrick consulted a woman named Christine Gerber who was channeling an Indian spirit guide named Marat. Marat said he was a 2,500-year-old spirit who had been a Seichim teacher in southern India.

It was Marat who told Patrick that the energy he was working with was called Seichim (Marat said the name as "say-chem" with an Egyptian pronunciation emphasizing the "s" and the "kh" or "ch" sounds). However, Marat was not able to translate his spelling for the name into the English alphabet because the "s" and "kh" or "ch" sounds of the Egyptian language are not a part of our language. This made it necessary for Patrick to create a spelling for the name. He wrote it several ways in his notes, and eventually settled on the name Seichim for a number of years. More recently, Patrick began using the term SKHM.

Over the years, other people have called the healing energy by various names including Seichim, Seichem, Sekhem and SKHM. This is in keeping with Patrick's later research into the name revealing evidence of an Egyptian hieroglyphic depicting a sceptre that translates as "Sekhem = s kh m" (see Part IV of *Her-Bak, Egyptian Initiate* by Isha Schwaller De Lubicz). See also the reference to the Sekhem sceptre in the *British Museum Dictionary of Ancient Egypt* by Ian Shaw and Paul Nicholson and in *Egyptian Yoga, Volume II* by Muata Ashby and Karen Clarke-Ashby. The pronunciation of the name has varied as well. Patrick pronounces Seichim and SKHM as "say-chem." Other pronunciations include "say-sheem" and "say-keem."

Marat also provided Patrick guidance on how to attune others to the energy stream. Combining this information with his Reiki training in giving attunements, Patrick began experimenting with passing the energy to others, including meditating and asking for higher guidance and assistance in his endeav-

ors. Several written accounts of the Seichim history mention at this point that Quan Yin, the Chinese goddess of compassion and mercy, came to Patrick in a vision and empowered him with the sounds, symbols and information for initiating himself and others into Seichim. Patrick indicated that his prayers for guidance did not produce such a vision. He went on to say that he had not even heard of Quan Yin at the time, making it improbable he would have attributed any of his experiences to her.

TOM SEAMAN

Patrick made three attempts at giving attunements before feeling he was successful with the fourth. It was shortly after this first success that he met Tom Seaman in 1984 at the Heartwood massage school where Patrick was both attending and teaching classes. Patrick recognizes T'om as one of the main links in the Seichim story. When they met, T'om already had received Reiki I and II from Phyllis Furumoto and Bethel Phaigh, two of the original Reiki Masters trained by Mrs. Takata. T'om was interested in Patrick's energy work and asked to be taught more.

Over the next few days, Patrick spent two or three hours daily teaching T'om both Reiki III and Seichim using the attunement method Patrick was developing based on his knowledge of both healing energies. Patrick also passed on to T'om a Seichim symbol revealed by Marat called Cho Ku Ret (more about Cho Ku Ret can be found on page 46). In the following passage, Patrick describes his work with T'om:

> T'om was one of the first to be initiated into Seichim. I held nightly classes where we shared energy and attunements. This was in a small community in Garberville, California. I had been working with Seichim for several years, and it was at this time I met Christine Gerber, who channeled Marat. Marat was the one who gave [a name to] the energy I was channeling.

Up to that point, it was only the most brilliant source of light I have ever seen. There was also an angelic choir-like sound connected to it. During class we would meditate and tone. On one of those nights, Tom Seaman came to class and asked to be initiated into Reiki [III], so I gave him the attunement. Then I asked if he would like the Seichim attunement with his not knowing what it was he had agreed to receive. He stayed not more than a week and we had a wonderful time together.

Not long afterwards he called me and told me he was having other symbols come to him. I assured him this was all part of the process. Later he also sent me a list of about 30 or more other symbols [the papers actually show 72 symbols] that were part of another language one of his teachers [a swami] had given to him. He experimented with those and eventually did not use them anymore. I had very little contact with T'om after that. Every few years he would call and we would update each other on our travels.

When I spoke with T'om, he shared with me his experience of learning Reiki, then meeting and studying with Patrick:

I wanted to share this [Reiki] with people, but I didn't have ten thousand dollars [the cost of a Reiki Master attunement]. I said a prayer in the back of my head and wrote Phyllis a letter [saying], "It is as easy for a rich man as sneezing but it is not that easy for me and I don't see the justice in that." And she replied, "If you are really meant for it, the money will come magically. It will drop in your lap." So I responded, "If it drops in my lap, then I want to pass on the energy to the people who could not or would not get it through the Reiki lineage." Over the next year or two, I continued to silently repeat my prayer.

One day in 1984, I was hitchhiking and got dropped off at Heartwood, which is a school of massage in Northern California. That is where I met Patrick. I had a friend who was teaching at the

school. While there, I talked to someone who said I should meet Patrick, and I did. Patrick had spent various times in his life doing different practices and meditations, so he was already well on the way and primed.

Patrick had been working with Christine and Marat and had tried to initiate others into teaching, and the first three times it didn't work. The fourth time it finally did ... with Christine. I was the fifth person along. Without any question of payment, we just started working and had this rapport. We spent a lot longer than usual and he had several of his students sit at the corners of the room and send support energy for the process. It was a wonderful experience.

After it was over, I said, "What can I give you?" and he said, "I have been starting to work with crystals" and asked if I had any with me. So I pulled out a 50-cent quartz crystal about the size of my thumb and said, "This is what I've got." Patrick was delighted and said, "Thank you."

After T'om left Patrick, he was excited to share what he had learned. He contacted his Reiki teacher Bethel Phaigh and declared, "I want to show you what [Patrick] showed me and see if it is similar to what you learned." Bethel confirmed that T'om's attunements with Patrick had included all of the important features of an attunement and would say no more, as she was sworn to secrecy as a Reiki Master. T'om described receiving further validation of Seichim as a healing energy as follows:

I had an acquaintance with a swami. I went over to his house and asked him if he had ever heard of Seichim. He said, "Oh, yes, when I traveled in southern India, I heard about that and have always wanted to follow up on it but have never had a chance. Tell me what you know." This was a confirmation. I also met a man at a retreat center in Oregon who had traveled in southern India. He said that while there he met with a healer who had kept trying to give him stones. They didn't have

any language in common. The healer kept trying
to give him a rock or two and kept saying words.
The only word that was consistent was Seichim.

T'om soon began sharing the healing energy with others, calling it Seichim. In general, T'om's teachings consisted of all of the symbols and information he received from Patrick about Reiki and Seichim, including Cho Ku Ret. In the first few years, T'om and some of his students also experimented with many other symbols. Some of these have come to be associated with various Seichim systems that are attributed to T'om as the originator. I asked T'om about these attributions, and he replied that he did not then, nor does he now, seek to create a lineage or a structured form of Seichim with a set number of levels and symbols. Over the years, T'om estimates that he trained more than 50 Seichim teachers. His classes typically have had one to three students at a time. He has lost track of the total of how many people have attended his Seichim classes.

In 1990, T'om's father became ill, making it necessary for T'om to spend most of his time with his family for what turned out to be almost ten years. T'om described this time as a period of great and profound learning. He also spoke of his experience as "benestrophic" (combining beneficial and catastrophic). During this time, T'om taught only a few classes, yet those who he trained as teachers have continued to teach others. Today T'om feels this decade-long period of being focused inward is ending, and another cycle of working with others is opening up.

PHOENIX SUMMERFIELD

The first two students trained by T'om as Seichim teachers were his swami friend and another friend, Faun Parliman. One of Faun's earliest students was a woman named Kathleen J. McMaster. Many historical accounts of Seichim use the name of "McMasters." However, I was able to confirm that "McMaster" is correct. Kathleen later changed her name to Phoenix Summerfield, which is how I refer to her throughout this Guidebook.

Faun first met with Phoenix in her home near Los Angeles, California in 1985. Phoenix already had received Reiki I and II and was interested in becoming a Reiki Master along with learning Seichim. Faun's spirit guides told her that Phoenix was not fully ready for the attunement yet also told Faun to proceed with it. Faun still had her own doubts and though she did give the attunement to Phoenix, she purposely did not pass on certain portions of the information about Seichim, including the symbol Cho Ku Ret.

Not long after her attunement with Faun, Phoenix located T'om and received from him the balance of the Seichim teachings, supplemented by later telephone conversations with Patrick. T'om saw that Phoenix was eager to create a standardized form of Seichim with levels and symbols similar to Reiki. The two also worked together for a short period of time on developing symbols.

Following her work with T'om, Phoenix brought in additional symbols and developed a seven-facet Seichim system that included the three degrees of Reiki. This is the form eventually passed to me and described in this Guidebook. However, with the exception of the Reiki symbols, Cho Ku Ret and a symbol named Shining Everlasting Flower of Enlightenment, I was not able to determine with absolute certainty the origins of the two other two symbols used in Phoenix's Seichim system (see the section entitled The Sekhem-Seichim-Reiki Sacred Symbols beginning in page 40 for more information in this regard).

Patrick credits Phoenix with being highly influential in spreading the word about Seichim by sharing the energy at expos and teaching many classes. Both Patrick and Marsha Nityankari Burack shared with me that Phoenix truly loved Seichim and considered teaching it to others as her soul purpose and life's work. She continued teaching until her death in the early summer of 1998. Patrick described his relationship with Phoenix over the years and his last conversation with her:

[When Phoenix first called me in 1987], she

expressed a great interest in Seichim and said she and T'om had added some new symbols. I expressed to her that she was free to teach in any way she felt guided. Soon she sent me a packet of all the information and artwork she had put together. At that time, she was doing lots of healing fairs and expos. I even did some artwork for her that she put on T-shirts. We got along very well and every few years, we would call and share our lives. I was raising a daughter and went through a divorce and she helped me through that time. I spoke to her while she was going through breast cancer.

Since then we spoke on various occasions. The last time was [in late 1997] right before she went into a nursing facility. Her spirits were high and she was really letting her child out. She told me she was having many requests for Reiki and Seichim and, of course, many wanted the final attunement. She could not remember how to do any of the attunements and asked me how to do them. I explained it to her as much as I could but reminded her that I did not do it the same way, as I did not use the symbols. She said, "I know. I don't use them either. I feel so close to Heaven now they are not necessary." There were many who helped her through this time and she wanted me to know that those are the people to whom she passed her light and love.

Though T'om and Phoenix had some philosophical differences in their approach to working with Seichim, he readily acknowledged her contribution of spreading Seichim around the world and described her work as a service to the planet. Similarly, Faun also recognized Phoenix's work for being important in making Seichim avail-

able to so many.

Through Marsha Nityankari Burack, I have been able to confirm that all of the Seichim information and papers provided to me by Seichim Master Sandra Koppe are either quite similar to or identical with the Seichim papers originally written by Phoenix and later given to Nityankari when she received Seichim from her original teacher, Barbara Van Diest, sometime in the late 1980s. Other Seichim information and documentation given directly to Nityankari by Phoenix near the end of her life as well as papers given to Patrick by Phoenix in the earlier phases of her work with Seichim also verify the accuracy of my own material. Nityankari was friends with Phoenix and is one of the earliest authors to publish information about Seichim in her 1995 book *REIKI: Healing Yourself & Others.*

One item of historical interest found in these papers is the Seichim logo developed and used by Phoenix, depicted on the left portion of the illustration below. This illustration came from a page Phoenix gave to Patrick near the end of 1987. According to Patrick, she worked with an artist to create this logo, then passed it to Seichim Master Teachers trained by her for use in their literature and certificates. This is the same logo I eventually received upon becoming a

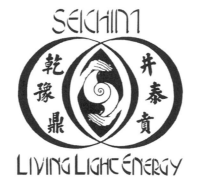

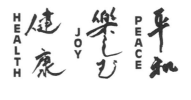

Seichim Logos: In addition to her legacy as a Master Teacher and Healer, Phoenix Summerfield also made very practical and creative contributions to the development of Seichim, including these professional graphics.

Seichim Master but by then, no explanation or translation accompanied it.

I was at last able to pinpoint Phoenix's original intent and explanation of the Seichim logo when Patrick provided me with an advertising brochure of Phoenix's dated February 1988. Within the logo, she described Seichim as "Living Light Energy" and called the entire logo "The Ovoid Symbol of Yin." The characters on the right and left sides were selected from the *I Ching*, an ancient Chinese oracle and divination tool. Translated from Chinese, *I Ching* means *The Book of Change*.

As depicted and described by Phoenix, the characters running from top to bottom on the left side of the Seichim logo are: Creative Energy, Harmony and Cosmic Order. On the right side of the logo, the characters from top to bottom are: The Source, Prosperity and Grace. The almond-shaped middle portion of the logo is Healing Hands Bringing Forth The Sacred Spiraling Energy.

My own research into this logo provides additional insight into its possible meaning. I could not determine whether Phoenix was aware of this additional information, but have included it here because it contributes additional clues to the meaning of the Seichim logo that she developed.

The almond-shaped area created where the two circles overlap is known in sacred geometry as a mandorla or vesica piscis. According to *An Illustrated Encyclopaedia of Traditional Symbols* by J.C. Cooper, this "'mystical almond' … depicts divinity; holiness; [and] the sacred … [and] also denotes an opening or gateway." Cooper goes on to say that all opposites and dualities are represented by the portions of the two circles that do not overlap. In *Awakening to Zero Point,* Gregg Braden further states that the vesica piscis is the Egyptian glyph representing both the mouth and the creator.

The two overlapping circles and the vesica piscis of Phoenix's Seichim symbol are also part of another symbol in sacred geometry known as the Flower of Life, which has been found depicted on the temple walls of many ancient cultures, including Egypt. The Flower of Life is usually represented as a pattern of nineteen overlapping circles within a larger circle and contains the geometry of all creation. See *The Ancient Secret of The Flower of Life* by Drunvalo Melchizedek for more information about this important symbol.

The right portion of the illustration on the previous page includes another design developed by Phoenix that she used in her Seichim literature depicting Oriental characters that translate as Health, Joy and Peace. In addition, the illustration shows the seal used by Phoenix on her Seichim certificates when her name was still Kathleen J. McMaster. Patrick provided me with still another graphic used by Phoenix (below) showing a prone human form being held between two hands. This graphic was printed on her literature in high gloss gold.

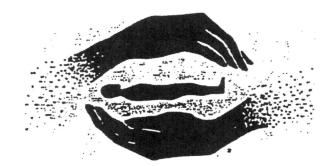

Healing Hands Graphic

PATRICK'S EVOLVING WORK WITH SEICHIM/SKHM

During the same time period in 1984 when Patrick met T'om, he also gave an attunement to David Quigley, the developer of a healing technique called Alchemical Hypnotherapy. Patrick went on to study with David for nine months, giving him a foundation in applying past life regression and deep emotional process work for healing himself and others. Toward the end of these studies, David gave Patrick the opportunity to assist in teaching several classes. This was a formative stage for what later emerged as Patrick's approach to healing with the SKHM energy stream.

Following his time with T'om and David, Patrick continued to work with the Seichim energy, including giving attunements to those who requested them. However, he preferred to remain in the background of the developing public interest in Seichim as a healing modality. Patrick left the United States again in 1985 to live and work in the Sudan for a year. Upon his return to the United States in 1986, Patrick enrolled in school for two years and completed a masters degree in architecture. While he was in school, Patrick taught three Seichim classes and then did not teach again until 1990. From 1985 to 1990, Patrick did his individual healing work chiefly with family and friends. Beginning in 1990, Patrick expanded his healing practice to include clients. It was at this time that he also began teaching regular Seichim classes again.

In 1994 and 1995, Patrick participated in an eighteen-month energy healing course taught by Robert Jaffe, founder of what was then known as the School of Energy Mastery. Patrick also attended two four-day weekend seminars facilitated by Brian Grattan, author of *Mahatma I and II: The I AM Presence*. The Jaffe course emphasized techniques for working with the shadow self, grounding the soul into the body and working in a group setting. The Grattan seminars dealt primarily with strengthening and grounding a person's connection to the angelic realms and the Source of ALL LOVE.

Both of these experiences gave Patrick additional training in facilitating others in the healing process and greatly enhanced his own personal healing.

As a result of these workshops, Patrick now understood the healing process more intimately and wanted to share this knowledge with others. He also recognized he had more fully grounded the Seichim energy within himself and sensed an inner readiness for the next phase of his work, particularly within a group setting. Patrick felt the information and skills he acquired in the classes taught by Quigley, Jaffe and Grattan greatly accelerated and enhanced the healing process and were an important adjunct to his work with the SKHM energy stream. He immediately began incorporating this wisdom into his approach to healing both in groups and with individuals.

Today Patrick teaches SKHM primarily in groups and works with the energy as guided, without breaking it down into symbols or facets such as those used by T'om, Phoenix and others over the years. Patrick leads a weekly SKHM group that has been meeting for three years, with various members coming and going during that time. In August 1999, he completed facilitating the first one-year SKHM teacher's training group in which I participated and has plans for more training groups in the future. In addition, he teaches SKHM workshops in the United States and abroad. Additional information on Patrick's current way of working with the SKHM energy stream is available in the section entitled Patrick Zeigler's Approach to Healing with SKHM beginning on page 26.

A newly-evolving aspect of Patrick's current work incorporates the last piece of information Marat gave to him in 1984—the use of what Marat termed the "breath of life." Patrick did not reveal this part of the information to anyone until recently because he knew that he did not yet understand himself what Marat was conveying. For many years, Patrick thought that perhaps the Reiki symbol Hon Sha Ze Sho Nen was the breath of life.

He knew without a doubt that he had found the answer to his questions when he came across a reference to the Egyptian ankh that described it as the breath of life (see Chapter 7 of *Symbol & Magic in Egyptian Art* by Richard H. Wilkinson). After this revelation, he more fully understood the meaning of Marat's conveyance. Patrick is now including this knowledge in his teachings to help everyone, including himself, integrate the energy of the ankh into all levels of their experience. See the sections entitled The SKHM Shenu on page 9 and the Afterword on page 111 for a discussion on the ankh and its relevance to SKHM.

Sekhem

By 1996, I was already both a Reiki and Seichim Master. I was teaching Reiki and Seichim together as well as operating a successful private healing and counseling practice in which I regularly worked with both energies during sessions. I was constantly being asked questions about each of the modalities, such as what they were, how they differed and how they worked together. Each time I was questioned by clients and students, I answered as best as I could, yet intuitively sensed there was much more to understand and experience with the energies. During meditation, I asked the same questions myself.

In June 1997, Patrick came to my area to teach a weekend workshop. I was excited at the prospect of having all my questions answered, since Patrick was the person who had brought Seichim to the United States. I arrived at the workshop full of anticipation and quickly realized the weekend was not going to be in a question and answer format. Rather, it was totally experiential with a bit of history-telling on the first day.

Patrick led us through meditations and showed us how to bring the energy stream into our hearts, minds and bodies. The Seichim energy did the rest. The energy led each participant to have his or her own unique experience. Some toned joy and some grief and sadness. Some wept and some smiled and laughed.

Some shouted to the rooftops. In the end, all present had been gifted with exactly the degree of the energy that they were ready and willing to accept and ground within themselves.

My experience of the weekend was profound. Though my questions had not been addressed verbally, they had been answered beyond my expectations through the experiential format. There was an immediate uplifting and expansion of the quality of energy coming through in my teaching and my work with clients. I also knew without a doubt from the very core of my heart that this energy and I were exactly the same. No longer were Reiki and Seichim something I channeled. I, myself, *was* Reiki and Seichim and much, much more.

The "much, much, more" presented itself immediately. I quickly realized that there was a third related, yet distinct, light energy coursing into and through me. I intuitively recognized that I had received a spontaneous initiation and opening into this energy flow as a result of the weekend with Patrick. I asked the flow about itself, and it said its name was Sekhem. In the next few days, new words and new insights came to me that described Sekhem, Seichim and Reiki and answered all of my earlier questions. I also channeled the Sekhem symbol, Heart of the Christos, during this period as well as enhancements to the attunement ceremony and teaching curriculum.

When I asked if additional symbols and facets were to come, the Sekhem energy answered that this was not necessary. The energy stream characterized its nature as being one to be held in a universal framework encompassing all traditions and heritages rather than narrowing it down to only one or two. Thus, terms such as Christos, Christ Consciousness and I Am Presence were to be understood in a universal context referring to a state of enlightenment and unity consciousness obtainable by all.

As I worked with this new energy flow, I came to understand and envision this ever-expanding energy stream in a way that had not been conveyed during my earlier Reiki and Seichim attunements and classes. Ever since this experience, I have taught all three energies together as SSR. I incorporated all three names into the SSR energy matrix for teaching purposes, yet know them to be as One.

The logo developed by me for SSR, shown to the right, combines the Sekhem symbol Heart of the Christos, the Seichim logo developed by Phoenix Summerfield and the Japanese characters for Reiki. The three are placed in a vertical arrangement with Reiki as the foundational Earth energy flowing into Seichim as the Heaven energy. Sekhem is the third element of the SSR trinity that unifies Reiki and Seichim as One.

A few months after the weekend Seichim workshop, I spoke to Patrick on the telephone and told him about my experiences and insights. He confirmed I had undergone a spontaneous initiation and shared more with me about his own experiences and observations of others who had gone through a similar opening.

Patrick also said that he felt in accord with my new understanding of the energy stream and encouraged me to further develop SSR. We laughed about how my questions had been answered with his saying hardly a word that weekend. We also acknowledged that we had each in our own way only just begun to scratch the surface in comprehending the scope of this wondrous and infinite energy stream.

The Sekhem-Seichim-Reiki Family Tree

I personally do not emphasize the significance of someone's SSR lineage because I feel the most important connection that anyone can seek to make is with the Source of ALL LOVE from which flows every form of interrelationship a person can have. However, sometimes people are interested in knowing the names of those who precede them in their family tree.

Appendices III and IV include a family tree or lineage for the attunements I have received for both Reiki

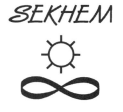

SEKHEM

Heart of The Christos

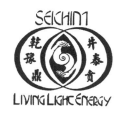

SEICHIM

LIVING LIGHT ENERGY

REIKI

Universal Life Force

SSR Logo: This graphic combines images from all three components of the Sekhem-Seichim-Reiki energy matrix.

and Seichim as well as one for the Sekhem portion of SSR that was channeled by me after my first weekend workshop with Patrick Zeigler. Each branch of the tree ends with my name. If you have received SSR attunements from anyone besides me, you will need to ask your master teacher to fill in the other teachers whose names would come after mine. Then add your name. Should you become a teacher yourself, many of your students and the students who they eventually teach will appreciate your attention to these details.

Other Seichim Healing Systems

Since Seichim was first introduced in the United States by Patrick in 1984, many forms of beneficial healing systems have developed around the world that use the name Seichim as well as other names such as Seichem, Sekhem and SKHM. They all have sprouted and grown from the same seed. It can be confusing, however, to both the newcomer and those who have studied some form of Seichim, because it is common to find multiple systems using identical names even though they can greatly differ from one another in form and content.

Therefore, do not assume that one Seichim or SKHM healing system is the same as another just because they share the same name. As well, the training and background of practitioners and teachers of these systems varies widely. Because of these differences, it is recommended that you thoroughly research all available options to find both a system that meets your needs and a suitable practitioner and teacher. With regard to the latter, please refer to the section entitled Qualities and Values of a Healing Practitioner and Teacher on page 82 for criteria to help you in your selection process.

Though it is not within the scope of this Guidebook to provide detailed information about every Seichim system that has emerged, they were all built on the foundation of one or more of the three distinct styles of working with the energy stream developed by the three key people who were part of Seichim's formative days as more fully discussed in the section entitled The Sekhem-Seichim-Reiki and SKHM Story beginning on page 11.

The first of these styles is Patrick's approach, which has evolved into working with groups and individuals. Though SKHM uses archetypal symbology such as is found within the SKHM Shenu, Patrick does not emphasize working with symbols like those traditionally utilized in Reiki. Further, although he initially employed an attunement procedure that was similar to Reiki, he soon shifted to other ways to help others connect with the energy stream. See the section entitled Patrick Zeigler's Approach to Healing with SKHM on page 26.

The second and third styles were developed by T'om and Phoenix. Recall that Phoenix was led to develop a fairly structured seven-facet Seichim system, whereas T'om's way of working with the energy was not focused in this way. Both healers experimented with additional symbols, some of which were created together. As well, both of their approaches to working with Seichim make use of formal attunements performed by a master teacher in a way similar to Reiki. Note, however, that some of the people who can trace

their Seichim family tree back to T'om have later created structured Seichim systems.

Today many more people are working directly with the universal SKHM energy stream and are channeling various symbols, adding levels or facets and creating new systems. Patrick has encouraged this growth because it is the nature of the energy to expand and express itself uniquely through each person who is touched by it. In 1997, Patrick answered requests for information on Seichim through a series of e-mail responses as follows:

I have not been ready to put out a document that says, "Here, this is what Seichim is." I have not yet been able to define it and hesitate to do so. Seichim is meant to be experienced and that experience is unique for each individual. There may be some overlapping experiences that many of us have and that is one reason why I teach in groups. It is truly my intention that everyone who attends a Seichim gathering will soar beyond any experience and expectation I may have had with Seichim and this is happening! It is so exciting to see others start with the seed of Seichim and create whatever they are drawn to do with the energy. Remember, there are no limitations, so why look for them?

The naming of the energy tends to put limitations on it. When I began to teach Seichim, the intention was for it to grow and evolve with each individual not dependent on someone else's beliefs, especially mine. It has done just that. Seichim has its roots in an Egyptian healing system as well as Reiki and both go back to Source. [Many healing systems have grown] ...out of the Seichim seed... I see it acted like a seed that has grown and produced many different varieties of fruit.

Some people tend to be attracted to the different varieties of fruit. I really do not see one as having more flavor than the other or the combinations of the different fruit as having the same flavor. The energy has evolved, is constantly changing and is evolving still. Those who have experienced what I have been teaching have noticed changes over the years. Originally Seichim was introduced from Egypt in 1984. It has evolved considerably since then within each individual who expresses it and then teaches it to another.

Some Seichim systems have developed to include divine guardians of the energy stream while others have not. In another 1997 e-mail, Patrick wrote his view on the question of guardians:

Many people who have been involved with Seichim have begun to have experiences with Quan Yin and other goddess energies such as Sekhmet and Isis. These have also been very much part of our group energy. For me, I have had some very powerful experiences with Horus. There have been times at a gathering where my vision would change and it was as if I was Horus.

I do feel these archetypal energies are within each of us and we begin to experience what is needed at the time. Eventually what is left is pure Source energy. It has no male, female or animal qualities. It just is. And as we begin to clear through the veils we find what is.

Seichim does not have any so-called guardians, it just is, though it is easier to experience the energy in a way that feels comfortable to us. If you are more comfortable receiving the energy from a goddess or god that is how the energy will approach you.

Marsha Nityankari Burack, author of *REIKI: Healing Yourself & Others* and a Reiki and Seichim Master, told me the story of how Sekhmet first came to be known as the guardian of Seichim in some Seichim healing systems. In 1992, Nityankari gave a Seichim attunement to a woman who worked in her office. The woman told her that immediately after having the attunement, she began waking up to the sound of a roaring lion. The woman researched lions associated with Egypt at the library and bookstores and came up with some information, including a postcard that had a picture of an Egyptian amulet with a lion's head.

Nothing else came of this experience until a year later when a man attended one of Nityankari's classes.

The man was very excited and said his reason for coming was to learn more about the vision of a roaring lion he saw when listening to one of Nityankari's audio tapes. He was also astonished that she lived in a neo-Egyptian style home that had depictions of the Egyptian goddess Isis and other Egyptian symbols on its outside walls.

In doing his own research, the man found Robert Masters' book, *The Goddess Sekhmet,* and passed the information to Nityankari, who came to an inner understanding that the Egyptian lion-headed goddess Sekhmet was the guardian of the Seichim energy. After Nityankari introduced Sekhmet to Phoenix Summerfield, she came to feel the same way and incorporated Sekhmet into her teaching curriculum.

One subsequent event further confirmed Nityankari's experiences with Sekhmet. When asking for guidance from Spirit about what the ruling energy should be for her Reiki center, she saw a lion. About a week later a woman from Egypt came to one of Nityankari's classes. The woman had in her possession the same gold amulet of a lion's head that had been portrayed on the postcard mentioned above. The Egyptian woman said the lion was Sekhmet and gave the medallion to Nityankari as a gift.

Since receiving my Seichim attunements, I have also had some moving experiences associated with various Egyptian gods and goddesses including Sekhmet, Isis, Bast, Thoth, Osiris and Horus, and a group of higher dimensional beings known as the Hathors, who are associated with Egypt and other cultures. I have found that the SSR and SKHM energy stream also seems to attract and be supported by many, many enlightened ones, some of whom may be identified and others who are recognizable simply as higher light beings who choose to remain nameless.

The strongest connection for me to date has been with a grouping of ascended masters who are a part of the Office of the Christ found on the inner planes, such as Jesus Christ, Lord Maitreya, Kuthumi, Mother Mary (who by some channeled accounts was Isis),

Djwhal Khul, the Buddha and Quan Yin. Most significant for me, however, has been the joy of welcoming and experiencing what has proved to be an ever-deepening and direct one-on-one relationship with the Source of ALL LOVE. An excellent discussion of these and other ascended masters can be found in *The Light Shall Set You Free* by Norma Milanovich and Shirley McCune.

Tapping into the Flow of the SKHM and Sekhem-Seichim-Reiki Energy Stream

The following describes two of the main ways of tapping into the SKHM and SSR energy stream that have unfolded since Patrick Zeigler first brought Seichim to the United States in the early 1980's. The first is Patrick's style of SKHM work; the second is through receiving individual formal attunements from a master teacher. Following these descriptions is a discussion about directly connecting with the Source of ALL LOVE, a third way of accessing the energy stream. Finally, additional comments about group work, attunements through a master teacher and spontaneous initiations are provided.

Patrick Zeigler's Approach to Healing with SKHM

Patrick works with the SKHM energy stream primarily in groups. However, most of the meditations, clearing and releasing techniques and other methods used in a group setting may be modified for working one-on-one in an individual healing session, whether in person or at a distance.

Patrick has used the SKHM meditations and practices in private for many years, both for his personal healing and to ground the SKHM energy more deeply within himself, and encourages others to do the same. Though the following discussion is centered on Patrick's group work, the reader will also find ways of applying SKHM both as a practitioner and for personal healing. It has been my experience that the healing process described in this section also applies when working with the SSR energy matrix.

Patrick's SKHM group work is currently organized into three formats. The first is an ongoing SKHM group that meets one evening a week, the second is a workshop format that usually lasts two to four days and the third is a training course for becoming a certified SKHM teacher. These groups are highly experiential and incorporate various techniques for working with the SKHM energy such as meditation, body movement, and sound healing through toning, overtoning and meditating using a gong.

Patrick's approach to working with others has evolved considerably, yet its core has always included three essential features: (1) an attunement meditation based on the information channeled for Patrick in 1984 through the spirit guide Marat about Seichim (see The Sekhem-Seichim-Reiki and SKHM Story beginning on page 11); (2) releasing and healing of physical, emotional, mental and spiritual energy blocks within the participants and himself; and (3) spontaneous initiation experiences. All three components are more fully discussed below.

Marat's information about Seichim included a description of a way to ground, harmonize, connect and attune a person to the energy stream. Patrick worked with this method on his own and began using it in every group gathering in a meditative format. The resulting SKHM Group Attunement Meditation found in Appendix V is not to be confused with the more well-known attunement ceremonies used by Reiki and Seichim Master Teachers (see the section entitled Individual Attunements from a Master Teacher on page 31) or with the attunement method Patrick used to pass the Seichim energy to Tom Seaman. Though the SKHM Group Attunement Meditation can be practiced while sitting quietly, the energy often inspires a more active experience involving body movement and sound such as toning.

Participants in SKHM groups also learn how to give another person a healing attunement. The SKHM Healing Attunement Technique is based on the Group Attunement Meditation and can be found in Appendix V. Patrick also leads the SKHM Infinity Dance during groups which can be found in Appendix VII.

These three methods are very powerful ways for connecting a person to the SKHM energy stream and stimulating the release and healing process. However, because SKHM is a flexible and fluid energy, the actual process within each of these methods can vary somewhat depending on how the energy is flowing in the moment at hand. Therefore, though each of these methods provides a basic template for accessing the SKHM energy stream, allow the SKHM energy to inspire and guide you as you make use of them.

Please note that the SKHM Group Attunement Meditation, Healing Attunement Technique and Infinity Dance have been included in this Guidebook to provide the reader with methods for connecting with the SKHM energy stream as tools for personal healing. Although the reader is encouraged to experiment with these techniques and hopefully will have a beneficial experience, Patrick has found that they are strongest and most effective when led or performed by an individual who has actively worked with the SKHM energy stream for at least one year.

This greatly increases a person's likelihood of having had a spontaneous initiation experience (see discussion below), which deeply grounds the energy stream into him or her. This grounding, in turn, greatly enhances the person's ability to assist others in activating the SKHM energy stream within themselves. As well, the person will have gained a greater understanding of the SKHM energy stream

and how to use it for healing purposes during the course of a year.

Patrick also feels strongly that a person desiring to teach SKHM in a group setting as discussed in this section must first develop many advanced skills for working with the energy stream both personally and with others. This requires study, practice, support and integration time of at least one year in a framework such as the SKHM teacher's training course (see the section entitled Teaching SKHM on page 91 for more information on this course). Thus, the SKHM Group Attunement Meditation, Healing Attunement Technique and Infinity Dance included in Appendices V, VI, and VII are intended to be used by the reader for individual healing purposes only. The reader is also referred to the companion volume to this Guidebook entitled *ALL LOVE FOR TEACHERS: A Manual for Teaching Sekhem-Seichim-Reiki and SKHM* for a full discussion of such advanced skills and methods.

Patrick has observed through facilitating groups and working individually with people that SKHM works with each person in perfect unison with his or her immediate needs and intention. This often involves first clearing from the physical, emotional, mental and spiritual bodies any negative, fear-based patterns and blocks that are lodged in the shadow self.

Moving beyond the fear can open up a person's energy system to create the opportunity for a spontaneous inflow of heightened initiation energy. Thus, it is possible for one or more of the participants, including Patrick, to have such spontaneous initiation experiences during a group session. For some, these experiences may occur in the hours, days and weeks following the gathering. Others may experience them much later, if at all. The intention, readiness and willingness of a person to receive and ground the energy at a higher frequency determines the timing of an initiation experience.

This is in keeping with the archetypal definition of "initiation" found in *An Illustrated Encyclopaedia of Tra-*

ditional *Symbols* by J.C. Cooper: a "return to the darkness before the rebirth of light." Cooper further states that "(i)nitiation usually requires a 'descent into hell' to overcome the dark side of nature before resurrection and illumination and the ascent into Heaven... ." While it is possible to access higher light frequencies without a so-called "descent into hell," doing so oftentimes can be a very ungrounded approach where the person leaves his or her body rather than truly integrating the soul essence into the physical vehicle.

As a person goes into the inner cave and faces his or her fears, the fear-based shadow material is emptied out of the energy system as well as from the body's cells and tissues, opening up space for the light to ground within the person. Prior to this cleansing and purification, the space is too full of shadow material. As long as there is even a trace of duality or polarity within the person, there will be fear present that must be cleared so that light can come to reside in that space. The clearing process is accomplished in an atmosphere of safety with the group's support.

Tom Seaman also described his experience of working with Seichim energy along similar lines:

This energy is an initiation into spiritual growth. It brings light into areas that might not have been gotten to so quickly otherwise. It brings up all your issues and your "demons." You have a choice between working through them and working them out or reacting, and acting them out.

In a 1999 e-mail, Patrick discussed additional observations he has made about the healing process that takes place when working with SKHM:

In working with the energy in its release and initiation form, I have found a pattern. This pattern is quite common in traditional emotional healing work except that in the traditional form, an initiation does not occur in most cases. Usually in the SKHM work, there are the following stages:

- *Identification*
- *Expression*
- *Release*
- *Integration*
- *Forgiveness*
- *Gratitude Including Possible Initiation*

In the identification stage, it is important [for the person seeking a healing] to look at the energy block and identify what it looks, feels, tastes, sounds and smells like. Once it is identified, then it can be given a voice, which moves the person into the expression and release stages. Sometimes the voice may not be so pleasant. Usually an emotion is directed outwardly to someone or to a situation outside the self. The key is [for both the facilitator and the person seeking a healing] to hold a place of love while this is going on and not judge the emotion being expressed.

Many times at this point, the shadow self will emerge and want to express itself. After all, it has been tucked away for a long time and it finally has an opportunity to express itself. Just hold a place of love and non-judgment. Once the shadow is engaged, it can create a polarity and the energy will feed it even more. In some cases this can help a person go even deeper. Here it is better to just hold a space of love and acceptance.

In some situations, I have experienced an almost demonic-like energy being released. Just hold the love. Once this energy fully expresses itself and is heard, the transformation to light can begin. Usually behind the "demon" is a frightened child.

Until the energy block has been properly and fully associated with the true source of the emotion within the person, it is quite common to project [the feeling] onto the teacher or someone [the person] loves and feels safe with. Sometimes it can be a feeling of love or it can be hate or rage. I do prefer love, and I do the best I can to hold a space of love no matter what is being projected. It is just part of the process.

Usually during the integration stage, the higher self will come in and a knowing and realization will come over the person that helps him or her better understand the emotion. In most cases, a person will come to the realization they are responsible for their own feelings and that usually through their own projections and holding onto past trauma, they are the one responsible, not really the person they are projecting the emotion onto. In group situations, each person plays an important role because we are indeed mirrors for each other. During the integration phase, a feeling of forgiveness will come over the person. This is not something that can be taught, and is a natural experience of the heart opening.

As the integration stage comes to completion, the next phase of gratitude will begin to flow, and the cycle is complete. It is usually at this time an initiation may occur which is very spontaneous. This is not something that someone else can give to another and truly is an opening of the heart from within.

By working with the process over a period of time—sometimes up to a year—usually an initiation will occur. Once a person experiences an initiation, they will then be able to fully support another through the process. Also, during an initiation, a person may experience symbols or images that may help trigger a deeper initiation or help someone else in the group through one.

Please note that Patrick does not use the words "initiation" and "attunement" interchangeably. By initiation, he is referring to a spontaneous and intensified inflow of high frequency subtle matter directly to a person from the Source of ALL LOVE, with no intermediary required. This is the purest form of initiation experience, a sacred baptism marking the inauguration of a new stage of empowerment. It is pivotal in bringing about permanent transformation of the person's consciousness and way of being, as well as his or her ability to ground, connect to and embody the Divine. The initiation experience grounds the person's soul at a deeper level within his or her physical body, making it possible to remember the soul's

blueprint and purpose. Patrick's Great Pyramid experience is an example of such an initiation.

It can be difficult to describe a spontaneous initiation experience in words, and it is common for a person undergoing such a process for the first time to declare, "*Now* I understand what you have been saying about initiations!" Because initiation experiences tend to be quite remarkable and noteworthy, a good rule of thumb in knowing whether you have undergone the kind of initiation experience that SKHM activates is: if you have to ask if it has happened to you, then very likely it has not.

Each person's initiation experience will usually contain symbolic information that is uniquely meaningful to him or her. In general, there can be a feeling of electricity going throughout the room when the initiation takes place in a group setting. The energetic vibration often begins in the person's heart as a wave of joy and love that becomes finer as it spreads throughout his or her body. The person may cry tears of relief or joy, laugh involuntarily or feel waves of ecstatic love and rapture. The person's inner senses may also be heightened in such a way that he or she sees visions of light, and hears, tastes and smells celestial sounds, nectars and fragrances.

Some people have described the urge to stand up as they experience the sensation of a lightening rod coming down through the crown chakra into the central light column and on into the ground. This can produce the experience of feeling extremely tall and having an energetic tail that has been equated with the vertical column of the ankh. As the body continues to vibrate, the lowest point of the sphere of the ankh comes to rest high in the chest and opens and grounds within the heart. Simultaneously, the horizontal bars of the ankh become established, sending a charge of energy down the arms and into the hands.

As one person in the group moves through a spontaneous initiation, the vibration can stimulate others into their own initiation experience. However, the grounding of the energy that begins in the group setting may take several hours, days, weeks, months or even years for an individual to fully integrate and comprehend. As such, in certain ways, having a spontaneous initiation is really *only the beginning* of the process because it takes time to grasp the far-reaching effects that such an experience can have on a person's life.

One of my spontaneous initiation experiences took place in the closing hours of a weekend workshop taught by Patrick in November 1998. The weekend had been intense and included much release work by myself and others in the group. Early in the second day, I had moved into a very tender and vulnerable childlike space. I felt like a newborn baby. While I was in this space, one member of the group held and stroked my head. I found this very nurturing and healing because it touched a place within me that was starved for this kind of "mothering" and loving attention. More group processing took place after lunch, which helped to stimulate my releasing a particular energetic block that I had been feeling in my solar plexus and chest.

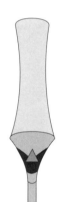
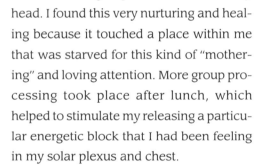

I happened to be sitting on a sofa as the release completed. Energy came streaming through my central channel into my crown chakra, making me sit up straight. My left hand was raised by the energy into a receptive position in front of my body. I could feel a golden scepter four or five feet long being placed in my left hand. It was similar in shape to the Sekhem sceptre depicted in Egyptian hieroglyphics meaning "Sekhem = s kh m" (see Part IV of *Her-Bak, Egyptian Initiate* by Isha Schwaller De Lubicz). See also the reference to the Sekhem sceptre in the *British Museum Dictionary of Ancient Egypt* by Ian Shaw and Paul Nicholson and in *Egyptian Yoga, Volume II* by Muata Ashby and Karen Clarke-Ashby.

My right arm was brought up high above my head with my hand and fingers moved into a salute, fingers pointing skyward. I felt myself sitting on a throne, and I was being coronated. I was greeted and welcomed as a member of a circle of light beings who were also sitting on thrones. This went on for several minutes. I felt hot and experienced tingling sensations. Simultaneously, I could hear the voice of my higher self advising me to sit still and simply receive the flow of energy. Throughout the entire experience, I was also spontaneously toning sounds that helped to open me up and ground the energy within my body. Other group members were holding my feet and legs to help with the grounding.

Since that day, my life has been deeply affected in many ways. The initiation prompted an immediate heartfelt forgiveness process that went to the core of personal issues surrounding my relationship with my parents, my siblings, others in my life, myself and, ultimately, the Source of ALL LOVE. I was able to literally go back through my entire life in a state of genuine appreciation, love and gratitude, making sense of each and every significant relationship and how each had played out and mirrored those unhealed issues.

Following this experience, I feel more deeply connected to my soul and higher self, the ascended realms and the Source of ALL LOVE. I am having memories of my earliest origins that seem to go back before the creation of the cosmos. I also received further expansions of my ability to channel and understand the nature of the SKHM and SSR energy stream. Further, I have become aware of my role as a gatekeeper of an interdimensional portal that opened to me in the hours immediately following the weekend through which I am presently accessing new information on the healing process, including a healing template that now seems to be an active part of me.

Though I am still in the early stages of becoming aware of the nature of this template and how to use it in healing, I recognize it is already doing its work inside those I am in contact with who are open to receive its blessings, all with little conscious effort on my part. I am hopeful that my ability to understand this template will evolve further over time. I also believe once such a portal is opened by one or more people, the information can be accessed by anyone who knows how to do so. Many people on the planet today are involved in such work.

Individual Attunements from a Master Teacher

Reiki is usually conveyed to a person through a sacred ceremony called an attunement that is designed to open the receiver to channeling the universal energy flow as both a healer and teacher of Reiki. These attunements are performed by Reiki Master Teachers who have received the same attunements and worked with Reiki for a period of time. Within the Reiki healing system, there are several attunement methods that vary from one another in certain ways, yet they each accomplish the same end.

There are three degrees for becoming a Reiki Master in some Reiki lineages. In others, the third degree is divided into two distinct steps. The first step usually includes receiving the Reiki master symbol. The second teaches the process of giving attunements for passing Reiki to others and in some lineages, adds additional symbols.

Most Seichim healing systems have also been passed to others through a formal attunement ceremony performed by a Seichim Master Teacher in a manner similar to Reiki. Recall when Patrick Zeigler first attuned Tom Seaman to Seichim, he used an attunement method that was based in part on his knowledge of Reiki. T'om then taught his students how to give attunements together with the related symbols and healing techniques. Other Seichim teachers who followed, including Phoenix Summerfield, further refined and modified the attunement methods used in many Seichim systems. (See the section on the history of Seichim/SKHM beginning on page 13 for a more detailed description of the evolution of Seichim.)

There are seven facets of attunement in the Seichim system that was originally passed to me. Other Seichim healing systems may have differing numbers of attunements. More details about the Seichim system that I first learned as well as information about SSR can be found in the section entitled Sekhem-Seichim-Reiki Practitioner and Master Teacher Attunements beginning on page 99.

Connecting Directly with the Source of ALL LOVE

Connecting with the Source of ALL LOVE is the goal of the two methods already described in this section, one achieved with the support of a group and the group leader, the other with a master teacher through an attunement ceremony. It is possible, however, to erroneously get caught up in believing that the group and the group leader or the master teacher and the attunement ceremony are an absolutely necessary part of the process, making your relationship to the Source dependent on them.

The highest form of empowerment does not require any middle person in order for you to directly access the Source of ALL LOVE. The spiritual development and growth work of each and every individual must necessarily include the development of personal responsibility for his or her own direct one-on-one relationship with the universal Source, with no middle person involved. Truly, this possibility exists for all of us and is a step we each must take at some point in our growth.

In keeping with this truth, there is a third way to receive the SKHM energy as modeled for us by Patrick, though it is not within the soul plan for most to receive a spontaneous initiation while spending the night lying in the King's Chamber of the Great Pyramid! You can simply sit or lie quietly in any place of your choosing and open to and receive the inflow of this divine energy stream assisted by various meditation and growth techniques used by the many spiritual disciplines available today. It is important, however, to remember to opt for a method that will actually ground the energy into the cellular memory of the physical body rather than encourage you to ignore the body and emotions altogether as some methods do.

You may also work by yourself with the SKHM Group Attunement Meditation used by Patrick found in Appendix V. Though it is fashioned for a group setting, make the appropriate adjustments and work with it accordingly. As I go through the steps of the meditation, I sometimes like to stand rather than sit and move my body in a slow spiral, keeping my feet in place and alternating in both directions. Next I move to patterning figure eights with my body, alternating in both directions, including my arms. I then move my spine in slow undulating movements from top to bottom and bottom to top to bring in the vertical column of the ankh.

As I work with the energy flow, I also consciously activate the horizontal bar and the round part of the ankh, bringing them together in the heart. I include making those tones and sounds that go with my body movements. In this way, I am incorporating into my body movements and the sounds I am making three key aspects of the SKHM energy stream and the SKHM Shenu: the spiral, the infinity flow and the ankh or breath of life given to Patrick by Marat. I find that doing this practice regularly helps to release and clear energetic blocks, further grounds and anchors the energy stream within my body and can stimulate additional initiation experiences. Doing the SKHM Infinity Dance found in Appendix VII can also produce similar results.

Another valuable practice would be to chant the mantra ALL LOVE while doing the body movements or as often as you desire during any of your daily activities. Meditating on the SKHM Shenu found on the cover is also a useful suggestion. See the section called The SKHM Shenu on page 9 for a description of the shenu and more suggestions on how to work with it for healing purposes.

Additional Comments on Groups, Attunements and Spontaneous Initiations

I have experienced all three of the preceding avenues for connecting into the divine energy flow of the Source of ALL LOVE. Each of them is valid and useful at different points in a person's soul journey. However, it is my feeling that as we evolve into living more fully as our true divine selves, the need for group support and individual attunements will become a thing of the past. Each of us will be able to freely and fully access any and all facets and frequencies of the universal Source of ALL LOVE as simply as reaching up and picking a ripe apple off of a tree. Some people are already beginning to do so.

Much of the value of either the group process or individual attunements comes from the clearing and release of old patterning and all forms of fear, which typically takes place during and after these experiences. A metaphor I like to use to illustrate this is to think of each person as a radio receiver that is trying to tune into the frequencies of the Universal station. Essentially, what each method does is clean up any static and interference (the patterning and fear) so that the Universal broadcast will be loud and clear.

These two methods also make it possible for a person to choose to receive and ground very high light frequencies of the energy stream over a period of time so that the physical and subtle bodies can gradually acclimate to the shift in the quality and amount of light being carried in the entire energetic system. These methods can greatly accelerate a person's spiritual journey and healing, opening him or her as an exceptional channel of the SKHM energy stream and assisting in preparing the way for spontaneous initiation to take place.

Working within a group setting or receiving individual attunements from a master teacher often provides encouragement and support to a person as well as instruction in different approaches for accessing the energy stream. The leader and the group or master teacher provide a "jump-start" that is intended to support and empower the person to apply what he or she has learned in creating a more fulfilling, direct one-on-one relationship with the Source of ALL LOVE.

I have also found that the ascended masters and an individual's guides and angels often take advantage of those times when a person actively opens him or herself (such as when participating in a group or having an attunement) as an opportunity to download information and guidance in accordance with the person's readiness, needs and prayer requests.

Another advantage of working with a master teacher and going through an individual attunement process comes from being given an established form in which to begin working with the energy stream. Patrick himself recognizes that becoming a Reiki Master after his Great Pyramid initiation was an important and necessary step in understanding the spontaneous initiation energy he received, integrating his many experiences while overseas and furthering his own personal healing.

As this process unfolded, Patrick was then able to define for himself his own perfect way of expressing and teaching what he was learning in his own unique form, which is still evolving. My experience has moved along this same path, and I am certain this is true for many others as well. As a person works more and more with the SKHM energy stream, he or she will likewise be inspired to expand and add to the system.

Some spontaneous initiations occur as part of our day-to-day living. Because SKHM is universal energy, it sometimes finds a person when his or her time of soul awakening is ripe, even if the person has never heard of SKHM. For example, only recently did I realize that some earlier experiences were clearly the beginning of my involvement with the SKHM energy stream. My first conscious spontaneous initiations occurred in St. Thomas (Virgin Islands) and Greece in 1982 and 1983, respectively, not long after I received my Reiki I and II attunements.

During the first of several spontaneous initiation experiences that took place while on these two journeys, I was lying down while in an altered state of consciousness for several hours. When I returned to a normal waking state, I knew without a doubt that my soul purpose was to be a vehicle for channeling and expressing Divine Love. The initiations that soon followed when I was in Greece further enhanced my healing and purification process and helped to prepare me for what later proved to be a full-time career in the healing and teaching professions. Other spontaneous initiation experiences took place in the ensuing years while I was on pilgrimages to Rome, Assisi and Medjugorje; while on a vision quest in Colorado and while visiting other sacred places such as Sedona and Mt. Shasta.

Spontaneous initiations also can occur during our sleep periods. Many, if not all people who are walking a spiritual path attend classes and gatherings on the inner planes and receive initiations during sleep periods. Though a person may not be conscious of these events, he or she will enjoy the fruits of these gifts during the waking state.

Both Patrick and I have also found that an initiation experience can be activated while simply talking with an individual in person or even while on the telephone. Many to whom I have given SSR healing sessions and attunements have experienced spontaneous initiations during and after our work together. It is likely that other practitioners and teachers have also found this to be true. As well, some who have come in contact with this Guidebook during its prepublication stages have also experienced spontaneous initiations.

The occasion for a spontaneous initiation ultimately cannot be controlled or planned, as the Universe in its infinite wisdom knows the right and perfect timing for each of us. Yet the more often a person chooses with intention to be an open and willing vessel of light and ALL LOVE, the more occasions the Source will have to bring such an opportunity to him or her.

Working with the SKHM and SSR energy stream is one of many possible ways of accelerating this natural process. A person may also work with various spiritual practices that actively invite the energy into his or her being in a grounded way. To create a balanced and holistic approach, it is suggested the individual also be actively pursuing his or her healing and growth process, taking care to consciously and deliberately attend to the needs of each of the physical, mental, emotional and spiritual levels.

One final matter about individual attunements deserves mention. There are two kinds of attunements used by master teachers. These can be thought of as "vertical" and "lateral." A vertical attunement is one that connects a person directly to the universal Source through his or her central light column. This column is one's direct line to the higher celestial realms and is anchored in the Heart of the Source of ALL LOVE. It also grounds the person and is secured in the center of the Earth. A vertical attunement builds, strengthens and expands the central light column.

A lateral attunement will connect the receiver with the universal Source, yet it also energetically links the person to the entire lineage of master teachers who have preceded him or her. It is my best understanding that this idea originated and became popular in some Reiki circles as a way to provide a form of group support and backing to the person receiving the attunement.

Though well-intended, my personal experience indicates that this can often create an undesirable energetic chain effect. The person who receives a lateral attunement must first energetically access the energy stream through all of the master teachers who are a part of his or her lineage and *only then* go to the Source to receive the energy flow. Because some forms of Seichim attunements were drawn from Reiki, this would also be true of lateral Seichim attunement procedures.

When I first heard of vertical versus lateral attunements from another Seichim master, I was mystified. It never occurred to me that I would be going anywhere for the energy except directly to the Source. However, one day as I was giving a combined Reiki and Seichim attunement, one statement in the ceremony stood out and struck me as possibly creating a lateral attunement. I asked for inner guidance and received confirmation of this impression. Soon after, two of my students made unsolicited comments that they felt they needed to think of me to get the energy flowing. This further confirmed what I was feeling about lateral attunements. I recognized that I also had been experiencing a similar kind of dependency on my own teacher that did not feel appropriate.

I immediately stopped using the statement in the attunement ceremony. Then I sat down in meditation and asked for all of the attunements I had ever received to be modified if needed so that they connected me directly to the Source of ALL LOVE. I also used distance energy work to redo all attunements I had performed up to that time to dismantle any unintentional lateral portion and replace it with a direct vertical flow.

The results were immediate. The attunement process was cleaner. I checked in with some of my students and found they were feeling a new surge of power. I felt much clearer as well, and from that point forward grew independent of my teacher and increasingly more empowered in my own right as a teacher and healer. The attunement method for the SSR matrix included in this Guidebook in the section entitled Sekhem-Seichim-Reiki Practitioner and Master Teacher Attunements beginning on page 99 reflects this deeper understanding.

PART THREE:
Healing with Sekhem-Seichim-Reiki and SKHM

The Heart of Healing

Opening the Door to Healing

On the evening of Sunday, December 16, 1979, I found myself quite uncharacteristically standing arm-in-arm as part of a circle of more than three hundred people in a dimly lit room. Our eyes were closed, and we were swaying side to side. Many were crying. We had all just spent the better part of five days together in an experiential personal growth seminar that turned out to be one of the earliest of many significant turning points in my adult life that put me firmly on the path of discovering and living my soul's purpose.

Though this was the first time I had ever participated in this kind of activity, I somehow knew I would never be the same. But it was not until the I heard the words echoing inside my head of one verse of a song playing in the background that I began to appreciate how profoundly I had been touched in such a short period of time: "Love is the opening door, Love is what we came here for, No one could offer you more, Do you know what I mean, Have your eyes really seen." *Love Song* was made popular by Elton John and its lyrics and music were written by Leslie Duncan (© 1969, Blue Seas Music, Inc./Jac Music Co., Inc., ASCAP).

As I listened to the rest of the song, its transformative message ignited the flame in my heart and I too began to softly cry. I felt both excitement and un-easiness over the prospect of opening up further to what I now recognized was still buried deep within me. Having unlocked the door to my heart, I could see and feel the love as well as the pain and the intense sadness and anguish that lay inside.

I also knew it would be much more painful to close down again than to move forward and continue the process of healing that had been made possible by my willingness to begin to take responsibility for myself and my feelings about my life. I had truly come too far to turn back.

And so began my journey into the world of healing. At the time, I had no clue as to what a healing crisis was or that I was on the verge of the first of many to come. I certainly had no idea of the many wonderful changes and transitions I would go through over the ensuing years as a result of that one single decision to follow the wisdom of my heart and learn to trust in love once again.

What Is Healing?

Within the sacred vessel of the heart lies the repository of your natural healing resources. The familiar expression "home is where the heart is" could also be stated as "healing is where the heart is." To heal means to make whole or holy. It can be defined as the process that reconnects and restores you to a wholeness and holiness that fosters balance, health and well-being at all levels including the physical, mental, emotional and spiritual aspects of your being. Healing is therefore defined within a much broader framework than simply addressing a physical or psychological symptom or attempting to cure a disease. In fact, healing is truly a way of life when held in this context.

Healing also includes your interrelationship with all that exists—other people, trees, plants, animals, birds, insects and places as well as the Divine. This interconnectedness creates a wonderful side benefit of healing: whatever you truly heal in yourself will simultaneously open up the same possibility for everyone, especially members of your family, who often share the same inherited patterning.

Keep in mind, however, that each of the souls for whom this is possible has the choice whether or not to accept the opportunity for healing. You need not do or say anything. Simply continue on your own healing journey and be a model to others of what is possible. This expansion of your personal healing also extends backward to your ancestors and forward to your descendants through your entire lineage, and includes your past and future lives as well. All of it returns to you in the flow of a circle linking the past, present and future as one eternal now.

Although many people have reported spontaneous healing of their health conditions or other imbalances, deep healing of the total person often involves a process that takes place over time. However, healing is not always a tidy, linear process. Rather, healing tends to follow a pattern that spirals and recycles over and over again, peeling away the layers of each issue until the healing is complete. This is because the original issue or symptom is most often related to more than one aspect of your life.

Your higher self will orchestrate the unfolding of each next perfect step in the process. For example, if you happen to be working on an emotional concern, you likely will discover a connection to your predomi-

nant thought patterns and belief system. This may next lead you to explore past life experiences that have a bearing on your current life situation.

You may then discover that your heart and mind are saying yes to healing, yet the physical body is strongly resisting. This is because the cellular memory of the body has been programmed for survival and protection based on the fear of change and past experiences of traumatic events such as being threatened, injured, dying from illnesses and being killed.

Oftentimes these stored memories come from lifetimes in which you were living in your truth and light while helping others to do the same, and were killed or otherwise threatened for doing so. When you begin reintroducing a love vibration into the physical body with healing energies such as SSR and SKHM, the body sometimes will translate it into fear because of earlier experiences. The cells of the body need to gradually learn how to let go of the old programming and trust and accept the new vibration of love and healing. The body must be reassured that it is safe to do so in order for healing to progress. This usually requires time, focus, patience and compassion.

In this regard, sometimes during a session, I have actually found myself engaging in a conversation with the client's body, saying words to the following effect:

I want to now talk with your body. This is a time of evolving and changing the fear programming that has served you very well and has helped you survive at times when this was necessary. You have done a wonderful job of protecting this person and he/she thanks you for this. However, as a species we are now evolving and shifting into a state of consciousness where we are going to be able to let go of the fear programming and live more fully in love. Our bodies will not be threatened anymore.

What needs to happen at this time is for you to gradually feel safe with this possibility. It's a whole new paradigm and way of being. I am introducing this to you right now so that you can begin to consider this and see how you might feel. Is this okay with you? (The client then listens to the body's response and answers. The conversation continues accordingly until completion.)

Healing also usually cycles through a series of discernable stages. The section entitled Patrick Zeigler's Approach to Healing with SKHM, found on page 26, includes a discussion of the stages of healing that he has observed when working with SKHM. I have found that these stages also apply to working with SSR.

Healing is most often a process rather than a singular event. I often liken it to putting together a puzzle. In the earlier stages of working on a particular concern, the person usually has only fragments or pieces of the puzzle that do not seem to be related to each other, fit together or make sense. As each piece is acknowledged one by one and dealt with using love, wisdom and patience, the overall healing picture gradually takes shape, allowing the beautiful mosaic of who the person really is to emerge.

The Healing Crisis

As you become willing to open each part of your life to the flow of healing energies and the process of self-discovery and growth, you very likely will come to recognize that you have outgrown old forms and beliefs. This will make it necessary for you to modify your lifestyle so that it is in alignment with your new perspective. While some parts of yourself may embrace and welcome such change, other parts will want to drag their feet and play it safe to maintain the status quo and remain in familiar territory.

Of course, life is filled with change whether planned for or not. Change signals that a cycle is ending and a new one is beginning. Life events such as the death of a loved one, the breakup of a significant relationship, losing your job, becoming ill, being in an accident or having financial problems are commonplace. Familiar and generally happier changes include getting married, having a baby, starting a new job, moving to a new home and retiring. Though some of these occasions seem to be created by outside circumstances beyond your control, they nevertheless arise from and mirror corresponding shifts and changes that are simultaneously taking place within you.

A healing crisis takes place when you are not fully and consciously ready for and accepting of whatever may be changing in your life. This creates resistance inside of you. The tension between what was and what is now coming into being influences one or more of the physical, emotional, mental and spiritual levels in varying ways.

Because the change is signaling to you that a cycle is completed, the natural flow of growth will become obstructed when you resist such change for too long by trying to cling to your old patterning and way of being. The more you resist and say no to the flow of life, the greater will be your suffering and the intensity of the crisis.

Though your familiar way of being is no longer viable, it usually takes time to let go of the old and move fully into the new. This results in your experiencing the void space and state of limbo that lies between the two. It can often feel like there is no solid ground beneath your feet. For some, these periods of upheaval and transition can be painful, chaotic, overwhelming, confusing, and filled with uncertainty and anxiety, particularly when you are not fully welcoming and prepared for the change.

Despite the challenges associated with change and purifying yourself at all levels, healing crises can mark significant turning points in your life. This is because times of crisis often provide the most fertile ground and tremendous opportunities for growth and healing. If you allow yourself to willingly, consciously and with courage go through the healing and cleansing process each time you are greeted by the need for change, you will find that significant growth has taken place especially over the long term. By releasing the past and learning to confront your fears and doubts about whatever is shifting in your life, you will open the door to many new opportunities for transformation and expansion.

The Purification Process Using Sekhem-Seichim-Reiki and SKHM

A great deal of purification and cleansing takes place as part of the healing process when applying the SSR and SKHM universal energy stream. Since SSR and SKHM both stimulate and support the process of healing and purification, it is important for the practitioner and teacher to inform each client and student about the healing process and be a part of his or her support system. Care must be taken to describe the process in a way that is thorough, yet does not cause undue worry or concern. The practitioner must avoid creating a self-fulfilling prophecy or expectation of always being in some form of crisis or drama.

As the SSR and SKHM energy flows through the physical and subtle bodies, your vibration is lifted as the energy works to align, balance and integrate all levels of your being. This usually involves the gradual release of physical, emotional, mental and spiritual "toxins" that have made their way into the cellular memory and built up in the energy system over time. Toxic buildup is the result of past experiences such as injuries, illnesses and traumatic events as well as poor health habits and pollutants in this and other lifetimes.

Much of the release experience is relatively gentle, does not take a great deal of time to work through your system and passes almost without notice. Sometimes, however, the manifestations of the cleansing process are more noticeable and uncomfortable and may take several hours, days or even weeks and months to work their way through your energy system. The cleansing experience is also heightened following an SSR attunement or an SKHM workshop because both of these greatly accelerate the healing and cleansing process.

As toxins are released from all levels of your being, you may experience one or more of the following symptoms of the purification process: The physical body may have flu-like symptoms, fever, headache, sore throat, coughing, aching joints and muscles, tingling sensations, nausea, constipation and/or diarrhea. Temporary changes may also take place in your sleep habits such as needing to sleep more often and longer and/or being wide awake when you normally sleep.

Deeply held emotions that have been repressed from earlier experiences such as grief, fear, depression, sadness, anger, fear and frustration may surface for no obvious reason. There may also be times when suppressed memories or other recollections surface in order to allow the body and spirit to heal. You may also feel empty and alone. Old and current behavior patterns and addictive tendencies found in the mental body may become magnified. You may also experience judgmental, blaming, victimizing and abusive thoughts. As the spiritual body is purified, your beliefs about life, religion, relationships, how the world operates and your self-identity may be shaken and will need to be questioned and revised.

All of these experiences are commonplace and are not usually a cause for worry or concern. They naturally result from the process of bringing higher light frequencies such as SSR and SKHM into the energy system in order to lift and transform the person's vibrations. They are nature's way of purifying body, mind, emotions and the soul, making way for higher levels of consciousness to be grounded in the body. Rather than being symptoms of illness, they can be viewed as signs of healing in progress. **However, if you have any severe or continuing physical or emotional reactions or complications after receiving an SSR treatment, please report them immediately to both your SSR practitioner and to your health care providers.**

As uncomfortable emotions and thought patterns from your shadow self come into your consciousness, simply allow yourself to observe and experience them without getting too caught up in them. Think of this process as a train where each of the cars is marked with an emotion such as sadness or thoughts of self-invalidation. As the train comes through your consciousness, just let it move along without stopping it and climbing aboard any of the cars. Acknowledge the emotions and thoughts as they pass through, then let them go.

Welcome your new awareness of those false and limiting beliefs that no longer serve you and have the courage to let them go. As the well-known expression says, "let go and let God" move and work through you. Allow a new spiritual foundation to be formed based on true wisdom, inspiration and understanding. Read uplifting books and spend time with like-minded people. Meditate and look within for your own answers. Do breathing exercises to bring the life force into your body. Chant sacred sounds. Remember to call on your guides and angels, the ascended masters and the Source of ALL LOVE for assistance as well.

You also will find it highly beneficial to surround yourself with a caring support system and take advantage of the many healing modalities that can assist you at a time like this, including SSR and SKHM. Both complementary and traditional approaches to your healing process may be appropriate if called for, including herbal remedies, chiropractic treatments, massage therapy, acupuncture, homeopathy, sound therapy, rebirthing, aromatherapy, flower essences, medicines, surgery and psychotherapy. Be sure to allow sufficient time for integration of the SSR process no matter what combination of approaches you choose to use. See the section entitled Preparing Yourself on page 62 for other helpful suggestions.

As you take full responsibility for your life, your body, your emotions, your thoughts and your actions, you will gain a broader understanding of the evolutionary process of spiritual growth that many are experiencing today. Each success will help you to know yourself at ever-deepening levels and to build trust in the process and a closer bond with your angels and spirit guides, the ascended masters and the Source of ALL LOVE. You will then be able to better anticipate and be in alignment with prospective transitions, making it possible for you to negotiate them with relative ease.

Some Reasons Why People Seek Healing

There are many reasons why people seek assistance with their growth and healing journeys using SSR and SKHM. All deal with some form of change. If one or more of the following examples resonate with a person, then he or she will find that SSR and SKHM are remarkable additions to a total approach to advancing the healing process:

1. The person is facing one or more life transitions, changes, challenges or healing crises related to his or her physical, emotional, mental and/or spiritual health; relationships; work life; financial status or any other meaningful area.

2. The person wishes to change his or her negative addictive patterns, reduce stress and take better care of him or herself.

3. The individual wants to experience more abundance, happiness, love, joy and fun, and less worry, anger, depression, sadness and anxiety.

4. The person has experienced the loss of a loved one, a relationship, a job, a home, health, a cherished dream, a pet or any other significant loss.

5. The individual is seeking his or her life's work and purpose and the ability to create his or her life from an inner-directed source of being.

6. The person wants to connect more deeply with his or her higher self, angelic guides, the ascended masters and the Source of ALL LOVE.

7. The individual wants to understand who and what he or she is on a deeper level and find ways to live his or her life from the inner spiritual core and essence.

8. The person feels there is something missing from his or her life and wants to create something that is deeper and more meaningful, and that ignites his or her passion for living.

9. The individual is feeling "stuck" and knows he or she has some internal housecleaning to do.

10. The person wishes to discover his or her creative

potential, talents, capabilities and spiritual gifts.

11. The individual wishes to cultivate meaning and enthusiasm in his or her personal and work life and find purposeful ways to make a difference and be of service.

Though each healing session is unique to the person and to the moment at hand, my way of approaching each of the above circumstances is the same. Since all problems really come from the same erroneous belief in our separation from the Source of ALL LOVE, they all have the same solution—to heal the separation and to know in truth that you are already completely loved by and are One with the Source. As *A Course in Miracles* says, "There is no order of difficulty in miracles" and "Love is the answer no matter what the question is." The *Course* also speaks of "many problems" that all have "one solution."

When working with SSR and SKHM, I do not separate the energies, using Reiki at one moment, and Seichim, Sekhem or SKHM the next. Rather, I work in concert with the person's higher self and guides and ask for exactly the right blend of healing frequencies to come through to serve the person's highest good at that moment in time.

The Sekhem-Seichim-Reiki Sacred Symbols

SSR as described in this Guidebook has a total of 11 sacred symbols that are used by a practitioner during a healing session to activate and focus the various healing frequencies in specific ways. The symbols are multidimensional and carry universal light keys and codes that go beyond the restrictions of everyday language as well as the conscious mind. The symbols also hold specific higher wisdom and knowledge that are transmitted and activated through their use.

The illustration on the next page depicts all 11 SSR symbols. Though they appear flat when drawn on paper, the symbols are three-dimensional and are in continuous motion.

In the chart below the symbols, the first and second columns list the names of the symbols associated with Reiki, Seichim and Sekhem as they were originally given to me. The third column shows the SSR facet when the symbol is received if using the original seven-facet SSR system that is more fully described in the section entitled Teaching Sekhem-Seichim-Reiki on page 96.

The SSR symbols activate healing in the physical and subtle bodies, help open and clear the central light column and enliven the unified heart chakra. Though all of the SSR symbols affect multiple levels of a person's being in many ways, it has also been my experience that they each resonate with a specific area of the human energy system. This impression has been confirmed to me through angelic guidance. These distinctions can be useful when using the symbols during a session, yet become most important when performing an SSR attunement (see the section entitled Sekhem-Seichim-Reiki Attunement Ceremonies on page 99). The fourth column provides this information.

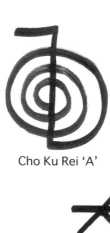

Cho Ku Rei 'A'

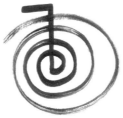

Cho Ku Rei 'B'

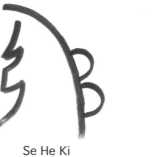

Se He Ki

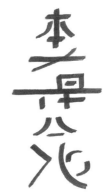

Hon Sha Ze Sho Nen

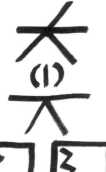
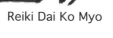

Reiki Dai Ko Myo

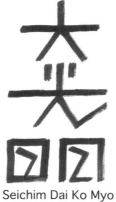

Seichim Dai Ko Myo

Cho Ku Ret

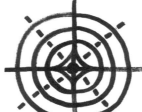

Shining Everlasting Flower of Enlightenment

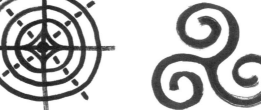

Shining Everlasting Living Waters of Ra

Shining Everlasting Living Facets of Eternal Compassionate Wisdom and Healing

Heart of the Christos

Energy	Symbol Name	Facet When Received	Areas of Resonance and Activation
Reiki	Cho Ku Rei "A"	Facet II	Physical including etheric
	Cho Ku Rei "B"	Facet II	Physical including etheric
	Sei He Ki	Facet II	Emotional
	Hon Sha Ze Sho Nen	Facet II	Lower mental (concrete mind)
	Reiki Dai Ko Myo	Facet III	Central light column to heart of the Earth
Seichim	Seichim Dai Ko Myo	Facet III	Central light column to heart of the Source
	Cho Ku Ret	Facet IV	Spiritual (higher abstract mind)
	Shining Everlasting Flower of Enlightenment	Facet V	Spiritual (buddhic)
	Shining Everlasting Living Waters of Ra	Facet VI	Spiritual (atmic)
	Shining Everlasting Living Facets of Eternal Compassionate Wisdom and Healing	Facet VII	Spiritual (monadic)
Sekhem	Heart of the Christos	Facets I-VII	All bodies + entire central light column+ unified heart chakra

What follows is a description of the applications and uses of each SSR symbol. It is important to note that the 11 SSR symbols work together as a unified whole, even though some were originally associated only with Reiki or Seichim. For example, you will use the entire SSR healing matrix and all of its associated symbols when sending a distance healing using the symbol Hon Sha Ze Sho Nen, which has been traditionally used only with Reiki.

The descriptions reflect both the original teachings given to me about each symbol plus additional meanings and applications when used within the SSR healing matrix. As you work more closely with the symbols, you will very likely receive additional intuitive guidance as to their purposes. See the section entitled Using the Sekhem-Seichim-Reiki Sacred Symbols on page 73 for further information on using the symbols during both in-person and distance healings.

Cho Ku Rei "A"

Cho Ku Rei "A" is the most frequently used symbol in Reiki and is known as the power symbol. It is used to incrementally increase the amount of energetic power being drawn by the practitioner during a healing session. Use of Cho Ku Rei "A" gives the practitioner the ability to turn the dial from low to medium to high. It boosts the degree of healing energy substantially and empowers and uplifts the energy level of the recipient. It also concentrates the power in the particular area that is being focused on in the healing work. Some other possible uses of the symbol include:

1. directing the symbol toward the walls, corners, ceiling, floor, windows and doorways of a room to clear the room of undesirable energies and to create a safe, protected space;

2. energizing lotions, creams, shampoos, medicines, vitamins, food and drink with the symbol;

3. relaxing the muscles during bodywork;

4. focusing energy and power into a specific area, place, situation or person for healing purposes; and

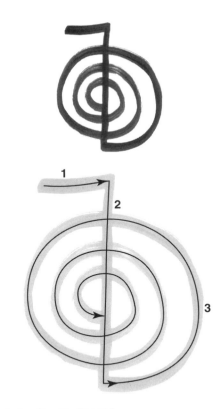

SSR Symbols: Cho Ku Rei "A"

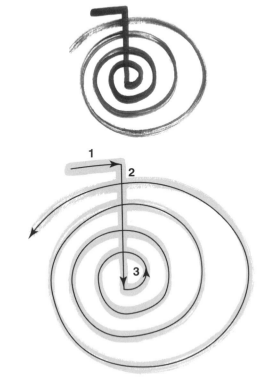

SSR Symbols: Cho Ku Rei "B"

5. creating a clearing, as with traffic, plumbing problems and finding a parking space. Use your imagination!

Cho Ku Rei "B"

The gentle action of Cho Ku Rei "B" assists with dispersing and releasing any form of negative energy and patterning being held in any of the physical and subtle bodies. Cho Ku Rei "B" is also good for pain relief and releasing stress and emotions that have built up within the energy system such as sadness, anger and depression. Like Cho Ku Rei "A," it is a counter-clockwise spiral, but it begins small and opens up to a larger coil as it moves toward the area being treated. This energetically opens the area, allowing the undesirable energy to be freed and released more easily. Another application of Cho Ku Rei "B" is in opening and expanding the chakras.

Sei He Ki

One use for this multifaceted symbol is as a protector from negative energies and influences. This protective function is especially valuable in helping to create an inner feeling of safety and security on all levels, including the psychological. In addition, the symbol may be placed around a car or used mentally to encircle a person to provide protection on the streets. If a person is particularly sensitive to negative influences from certain types of visuals such as may be found in television or films, the symbol may be used to guard against these kinds of intrusions.

Sei He Ki also helps to untangle constrictions and blocks that inhibit the free flow of energy in the same way that a comb untangles hair. Some like to visualize it as a dragon helping to untangle blocks with its fiery breath.

Boxing or circling Sei He Ki in a counterclockwise movement after first drawing the basic symbol is particularly useful for calming another person or yourself. Both the box and the circle used with Sei He Ki pull together scattered energy and create an energetic

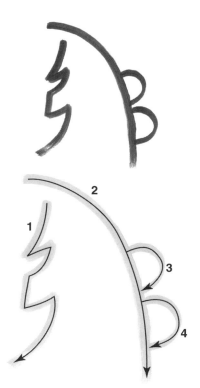

SSR Symbols: Sei He Ki

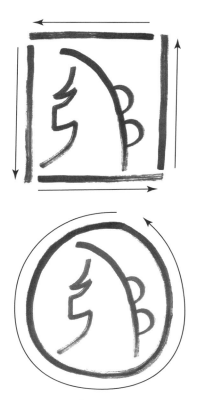

SSR Symbols: Bounding Sei He Ki in a counterclockwise box or circle helps with centering.

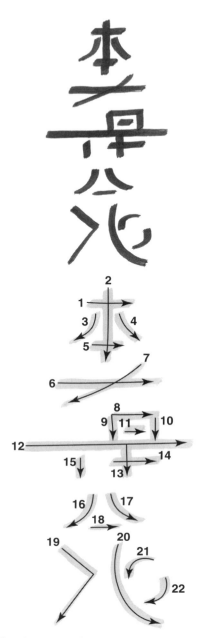

SSR Symbols: Hon Sha Ze Sho Nen

the cellular memory. Please refer to the section entitled Using the Sekhem-Seichim-Reiki Sacred Symbols on page 73 for a description of the technique.

Hon Sha Ze Sho Nen

Hon Sha Ze Sho Nen is the symbol used for absent sessions or distance healing and is a gateway that bridges time and space. Hon Sha Ze Sho Nen can be applied to anything conceivable including sending a healing to yourself for personal healing. You can send SSR energy to a situation or circumstances within a person's current lifetime or to ones that grew from a past life. You can also send healing to relationships, as well as to the past, present and future spiritual essence of a person.

While in-person sessions may last an hour or more, distance healings can be completed in substantially less time, even just a few moments. Instructions for sending a distance healing can be found in the section entitled Using the Sekhem-Seichim-Reiki Sacred Symbols on page 72.

Reiki Dai Ko Myo and Seichim Dai Ko Myo

Reiki Dai Ko Myo is the master symbol for Reiki. Dai Ko Myo means "Great Shining Everlasting Light." According to William Rand, two other translations are "Great Beings of the Universe, shine on me, be my friend" and "The treasure house of the great beaming light." Reiki Dai Ko Myo is used when giving a healing and, as the teaching symbol for Reiki, when passing attunements. The electromagnetic frequencies of all the Reiki symbols and the entire Reiki spectrum are contained in this symbol, yet it does not replace the need for using the other Reiki symbols when so guided. In fact, receiving Reiki Dai Ko Myo enables a person to open to newer and deeper understandings of all of the symbols in the Reiki frequency range.

Within the SSR matrix, the base color of Reiki Dai Ko Myo is rose pink, i.e., red physical energy that has integrated and blended with higher light frequencies

boundary that helps to contain and center a person. Using a box adds a grounding effect; using a circle calms and uplifts. This procedure can also be used for personal protection and to enhance the security of objects such as a car, stereo or house.

A profound application of Sei He Ki during a healing session is for releasing and reprogramming of physical, mental and emotional patterns found within

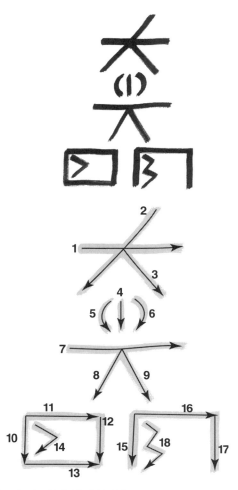

SSR Symbols: Reiki Dai Ko Myo

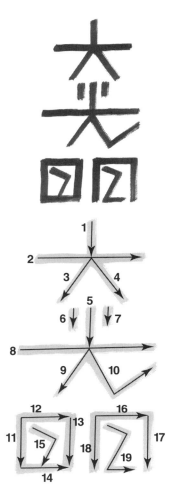

SSR Symbols: Seichim Dai Ko Myo

to produce rose pink. This symbol is the ground and anchor for the SSR healing system and for all forms of activities while living in the third dimension. It also opens the central light column, or antakarana, from the heart chakra through the lower three chakras and down into the center of the Earth.

The base color of Seichim Dai Ko Myo is electric blue, the same color of the energy that Patrick Zeigler experienced in the Great Pyramid. This symbol opens the central light column from the heart chakra up through the various dimensional levels all the way to the Source of ALL LOVE. As the Reiki and Seichim Dai Ko Myo energies work to open the chakras and the central channel, they blend and merge, bringing together Earth and Heaven in a perfectly balanced state of Oneness within the unified heart chakra (see the

section entitled The Unified Heart Chakra on page 4).

In Reiki Dai Ko Myo, the top character represents humankind in the third dimension. The second character represents enlightened humankind. The base of the symbol depicts shifting from one level of consciousness to another. The lefthand character of the base is the "illusion of a closed universe foundation" and on the right, the character is the "reality of an open, limitless foundational universe." The lefthand base character operates within the foundational realm, i.e., our third dimensional consciousness while in a physical body. Here we are taught a closed illusionary belief system which often trains us to believe that we are only bodies, death is real and there is no reality beyond what we experience with the five senses of sight, hearing, taste, touch and smell.

The shift in consciousness represented by the character on the right of the base breaks the spell of the illusion. The person begins to open to the reality that he or she is more than a physical body and asks such questions as, "Who am I?" and "What is my divine purpose?" However, even though the consciousness level has opened dramatically, the person is still operating primarily within the foundational universe and does not yet fully grasp the vastness and limitlessness that are paradoxically both a part of and beyond the third dimensional level of perception. Reiki Dai Ko Myo moves a person toward his or her divine nature within the heart chakra, clearing the way for Seichim Dai Ko Myo to do its work.

The first character of Seichim Dai Ko Myo represents humankind in the third dimension, while its second character illustrates "enlightened humankind kicking off to greater experiences." The base characters are two portals that represent two additional levels of consciousness beyond those described as part of Reiki Dai Ko Myo. The lefthand character opens the "doorway to the universe limited" and the character on the right opens the "doorway to the universe limitless."

When a person steps beyond the foundational universe opened by Reiki Dai Ko Myo, he will initially find himself at the doorway to the universe limited, because the ability to perceive himself into infinity is not yet fully accessible. His consciousness is still vacillating between dimensional levels. Ultimately, however, this vacillating stabilizes and the person is able to "kick off to greater experiences" as he moves through the doorway to the universe limitless and into the full realization of himself as an enlightened multidimensional being.

Cho Ku Ret

Cho Ku Ret is the symbol that was revealed to Patrick Zeigler by Marat as described in the section recounting the history of Seichim on page 16. Marat described the symbol as combining a spiral and the infinity symbol. Marat also defined the phrase "Cho Ku" as

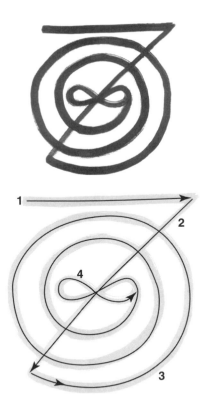

SSR Symbols: Cho Ku Ret

meaning "from the root or source" and "Ret" as meaning infinity. Therefore, the two combined as "Cho Ku Ret" means "from the root or source to infinity." Cho Ku Ret can be thought of as the bridge connecting the spiraling foundational energy of Reiki to the infinity pattern of Seichim. Within this symbol is the meeting place of Heaven and Earth. Further information about the meaning of the infinity pattern can be found in the section that discusses the SSR symbol Heart of the Christos.

The illustration above depicts the design of Cho Ku Ret as it was given to me. The illustration on the opposite page is an alternative version used by some practitioners. The SKHM Shenu includes the infinity sign and the spiral drawn in yet another possible way. Experiment with each version and work with the one that feels best.

This powerful symbol works interdimensionally, allowing communication on all levels and the ability to access all dimensions. It dissolves barriers to the higher self, transcending space and time and pulling

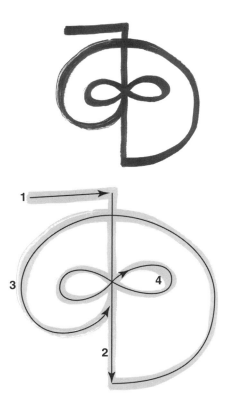

SSR Symbols: Cho Ku Ret (another version)

back the veil or curtain to the soul. By clearing away all blockages, the individual is able to use the interdimensional gateway opened by Cho Ku Ret to connect, communicate and channel information from his or her higher self or soul, spirit guides, the angelic realms, the Akashic Records and the ascended masters, as well as the Source of ALL LOVE. This symbol may also be used to facilitate communication with the plant, animal and mineral kingdoms and with nature devas, gnomes and fairies.

Cho Ku Ret works best for interdimensional communication when the central light column is open and clear. It is therefore suggested that Cho Ku Ret be coupled with Reiki Dai Ko Myo and Seichim Dai Ko Myo for this purpose.

In addition, Cho Ku Ret may be used with intention to activate the empowerment of objects such as crystals to support healing as well as for creating and manifesting that which is desired in a person's life.

This symbol is like having a special lens for a wonderful camera. If the camera symbolizes having full power and information, the lens allows you to focus that power for a specific purpose.

For example, you can empower a crystal with Cho Ku Ret together with a specific intention such as, "My relationship with my mother is healed," "I have a new computer," or "I have a successful healing practice." To do this, hold the crystal and invoke Cho Ku Ret and whatever other SSR symbols you are guided to use. Then send the symbols and your intention into the crystal until it feels completely charged. You can strengthen your intention by writing the specific purpose on paper and placing it and the crystal in a sacred place such as on an altar. In most situations, this is all you will need to do. However, in more complex situations it may be necessary to occasionally check in to see if the crystal requires clearing and recharging. You may also need to clarify and reinforce your intention.

Draw the symbol as shown by the arrows and numbers. Draw the infinity sign at the center of the symbol at least three times.

Shining Everlasting Flower of Enlightenment

This symbol was created together by Phoenix and Tom Seaman. Phoenix called the symbol Shining Everlasting Flower of Enlightenment while T'om called it Mayooora. T'om adopted this name after being told by a psychic that "Mayooora" was the sound the symbol makes when invoked. Phoenix's paperwork also indicates that she sometimes used the name of Mayourma which is very similar to T'om's name. In addition, T'om's version did not include the two Cho Ku Ret symbols on either side.

This multidimensional symbol shifts the energy center of the heart upward into manifestation. It activates and anchors the Christ Consciousness into the physical and subtle bodies and opens the person to

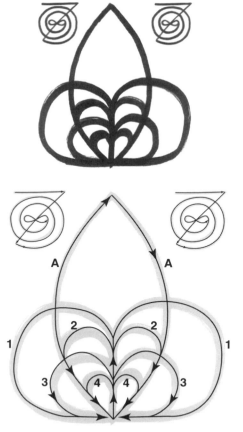

SSR Symbols: Shining Everlasting Flower of Enlightenment

1. With the right hand, draw "A" starting at the bottom center of "A" and circling around in a clockwise direction.

2. Draw the petals with both hands from either larger to smaller or smaller to larger. If drawing them from larger to smaller, start at the center of the petals and move outward, then back around to the center in the following order:

(Left hand)	(Right hand)
Petal 1	Petal 1
Petal 2	Petal 2
Petal 3	Petal 3
Petal 4	Petal 4

   If going from smaller to larger, start at the center of the petals and move outward, then back around to the center in the following order:

(Left hand)	(Right hand)
Petal 4	Petal 4
Petal 3	Petal 3
Petal 2	Petal 2
Petal 1	Petal 1

3. Draw two Cho Ku Ret symbols to the left and right of the upper portion of the flower.

Phoenix Summerfield's paperwork gave me insight into how she taught others to draw this symbol. The portion marked "A" is drawn first, with both hands starting at the top center, then moving down to bottom center. The dominant hand is to then draw the petals at the bottom of the flower in one continuous motion from the point at the bottom of the portion marked "A." In effect, this is drawing four infinity patterns of differing sizes, as shown in the illustration, to create the flower petals. The two Cho Ku Ret symbols to the left and right of the upper portion of the flower are then added.

Another way to use this symbol that was taught by Phoenix is to build an even larger flower by repeating the symbol four times as shown on the opposite page. This will magnify the power and effects of this symbol many times over.

allow and accept balanced love into his or her life. It dissolves barriers that have shrouded the emotional body and heart center, empowering an individual to manifest unconditional love and his or her deepest heart's desires.

Shining Everlasting Flower of Enlightenment also helps a person to access his or her soul blueprint and higher purpose. The symbol aids in transforming crises into meaningful lessons and accelerates the process of making prosperity, health and satisfying personal relationships a reality. Life begins to unfold as fast as the person is able to run with it.

This symbol can be drawn in two ways. Either way works well so choose the one that you like best. When I first learned this symbol, I was instructed to draw it as follows:

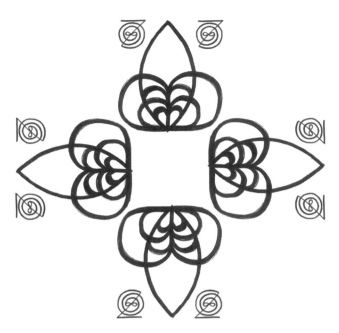

SSR Symbols: Shining Everlasting Flower of Enlightenment (magnified)

Shining Everlasting Living Waters of Ra

This multidimensional symbol embodies the two elements of fire (evoked by Ra, the Egyptian Sun God) and water. Though seemingly in conflict, fire and water are necessary for life as heat and moisture. In *An Illustrated Encyclopaedia of Traditional Symbols*, J.C. Cooper describes fire and water as representing the two great active and passive principles of the universe, including the "Sky Father and the Earth Mother and all the opposites in the elemental world." Yet as fire and water penetrate one another and become burning water, they join together in the union of opposites that is beyond all forms of polarity and duality consciousness.

The cross portion of the symbol also represents the union of Heaven and Earth, with the axis point being the Source of ALL LOVE from which emanates infinite spiritual expansion in all directions. The curved, web-like portion forming the Living Waters of Ra signifies the unification and consolidation of all powers into one central core.

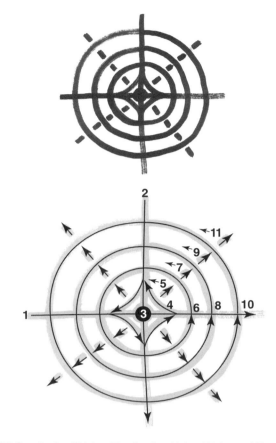

SSR Symbols: Shining Everlasting Living Waters of Ra

The fire and water elements that together form this symbol work in concert to clear and balance. The fire burns away, purifies and releases toxins and pains at the physical, emotional, mental and spiritual levels. The water at the center represents the liquid equivalent of light and helps dissolve and wash away the deep negative patterning found within these levels and in the cellular memory. As the clearing takes place, the Living Waters infuse the energy system with higher light frequencies, facilitating the union of the many opposites within the person. A synergistic balancing, integration and unification of the physical, emotional, mental and spiritual levels are also stimulated and the now-emerging whole person becomes greater than the sum of his or her parts.

The symbol can also be applied to seal an auric leak and to close the energy field at the end of a session. As well, the symbol can be used for protection whenever needed.

Two descriptions of the Living Waters of Ra found in Phoenix Summerfield's materials give further insight into how she envisioned the symbol. The first note describes "three dimensional flaming water spheres within spheres infinitely vibrating inward and outward"; the second states that "I visualize this as a pebble that drops in still water."

Because of its shape, the symbol further lends its interpretation to the symbology of the medicine wheel used in many Native American traditions. The medicine wheel includes the cycle of life, and the four directions, elements and seasons.

The symbol is also deeply connected with the heart and resembles the unified heart chakra, with the layers moving out from the center representing the physical body and each of the subtle bodies.

Finally, another perspective on this symbol was suggested by Tom Seaman when I showed it to him. Upon seeing this symbol, he said it reminded him of looking down from above on the crown chakra. From this viewpoint, the dot in the middle becomes the central column while the surrounding portions of the symbol depict the ways in which the energy expands into the various levels of the auric field. T'om also indicated he had not been a part of creating this symbol and that this was the first time he had ever seen it.

The instructions for how to draw the symbol Shining Everlasting Living Waters of Ra are as follows:

1. Draw the horizontal line of the cross moving from left to right (1). Next draw the vertical line, moving from top to bottom (2). Then place a small dot in the axis of the cross (3).

2. Starting at the three o'clock position and going counterclockwise, draw the four slightly curved lines (4). These enclose and represent the waves of the Living Waters of Ra.

3. Starting at the two o'clock position and going counterclockwise, draw the four marks within each quarter outside of the curved lines (5).

4. Starting at the three o'clock position and going counterclockwise, draw the innermost circle (6).

Now draw the next set of four marks just outside of this circle (7). See the marks and the circle ignited in fire.

5. Repeat step 4 at least two more times making each successive circle and set of marks larger than the last to encompass everything already drawn (8), (9), (10), (11).

Shining Everlasting Living Facets of Eternal Compassionate Wisdom and Healing

The top illustration on the opposite page shows the Seichim Master symbol as it was originally given to me. It is the universal key for all other symbols in the Seichim frequency range because the energy and power of all other Seichim symbols are contained within it. This does not eliminate the individual value of the other Seichim symbols. Receiving this symbol enables a person to open to newer and deeper understandings of all of the symbols that make up the Seichim frequency range.

The symbol can be traced back to pagan times and was quietly adopted after the rise of Christianity. Today it can be found on Romanesque church carvings and gravestones. Known as the "triskele" (from the Greek word "triskelion," meaning three-legged), this symbol is common to all six nations of the Celtic realm. The Celtic version is the lower illustration on the opposite page. The paperwork of Phoenix Summerfield contains this Celtic version and includes a notation that says, "May the holy breath fill you now." However, it is not known how Phoenix came to adopt this symbol as the Seichim master symbol.

The three legs or branches of the symbol are curved, radiating out from the center or Source and representing the trinity cycle of birth, death and rebirth. As discussed earlier, a trinity is distinguished from a triad as a unity; a three-in-one and a one-in-three (see the section entitled What is Sekhem-Seichim-Reiki and What Are Its Benefits? on page 7). This symbolizes unity in

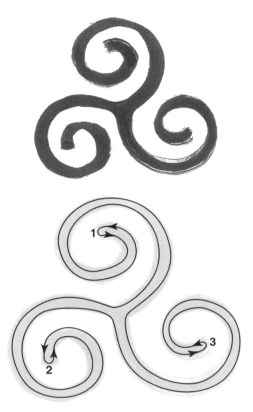

SSR Symbols: Shining Everlasting Living Facets of Eternal Compassionate Wisdom and Healing

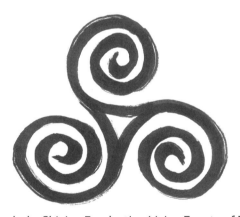

SSR Symbols: Shining Everlasting Living Facets of Eternal Compassionate Wisdom and Healing Celtic version

The symbol can be used in many ways, such as rotating it through a chakra or down the central light column for cleansing, breaking up and dissolving blockages and psychic sludge. It can also be used for balancing the chakras and widening the central light column. It is a universal globe form for encoding, instilling, programming and activating light languages and codes, mantras and other sacred symbols within the human form as well as within crystals and stones. It is a platform for assisting a person in resolving and rising above karmic issues so that the soul can move off the karmic wheel, integrate higher dimensional levels and move into full enlightenment. Moving off the karmic wheel is equivalent to being in total Oneness and living full-time in the energy of Sekhem.

Shining Everlasting Facets of Eternal Compassionate Wisdom and Healing is a symbol that can be used as a platform for accessing various dimensional frequencies, including other systems of healing. To accomplish this, the symbol sits spinning on a column while its arms move out to locate and access the appropriate dimensional frequencies. These are then transmitted from these levels through the practitioner for the benefit of the recipient. This process can happen spontaneously or be consciously invoked. The preceding visual description of how the symbol accesses other frequencies and systems of healing was channeled by Andrea Bowman, an SSR Master Teacher.

Similarly, the shape and the vibrational rhythm and qualities of this symbol can also be used to take a person into deep altered states of consciousness and then to bring him or her back to normal waking consciousness. Repetition of the process of going back and forth between dimensions gradually helps the person to further develop the ability to maintain conscious awareness of all dimensions and states of consciousness simultaneously.

To draw Shining Everlasting Facets of Eternal Compassionate Wisdom and Healing, move first from point 1 to point 2, second from point 2 to point 3, and third from point 3 to point 1.

diversity, with the third uniting the opposites. In the case of Shining Everlasting Living Facets of Eternal Compassionate Wisdom and Healing, the unifying leg or branch is rebirth, and the opposites are birth and death. Other examples include the Christian trinity of Father, Son and Holy Spirit and the Egyptian trinity of Father (Osiris), Mother (Isis) and Son (Horus).

Heart of the Christos

Heart of the Christos or Heart of the Christ is the name of the sacred master symbol for the entire SSR healing matrix and for all seven facets of Sekhem. Receiving this symbol enables a person to open to a greater awareness and understanding of the entire SSR healing matrix and the SKHM energy stream. This symbol was channeled by me in 1997 after my first weekend workshop with Patrick Zeigler and is not a part of the original Seichim system developed by Phoenix Summerfield.

"Christos" comes from the Greek language and means "The Anointed One." Though usually associated with the Christian religion, the terminology is used in connection with this symbol in its universal sense. It denotes the entire spectrum of higher light frequencies associated with embodying the Divine within ourselves through the process of ascension. In this context, Jesus Christ is one of a countless number of ascended masters who are working on the inner planes to teach us about this opportunity for soul evolution.

Heart of the Christos opens the lotus blossom of the heart to the indwelling Christ Consciousness and the I Am Presence. This activates, stimulates and further refines the ongoing process of balancing and integrating the physical, emotional, mental and spiritual bodies; unifying all polarities; and developing the unified heart chakra. Within the Heart of the Christos are the Love, Light, Power, Grace and Wisdom of All That Is. It is the Source. It is Home. It is ALL LOVE.

SSR Master Teacher, C.D. Stoune, describes a vision he had of Heart of the Christos during a channeling session not long after receiving the SSR attunements:

> The symbol is active and alive, and full of color and sound vibrations that pass through many, many dimensions simultaneously, including time. I saw the infinity symbol being illuminated from above by the central light of the universal divine emanating from the Central Sun. At the same time,

SSR Symbols: Heart of the Christos

> the infinity symbol seemed to be illuminated from within. As it spun and turned through many dimensions, the energy from the Central Sun pulsed through the winding curves of its figure-eight shape. It was all very colorful and vibrant.

In the original seven-facet SSR system, this Sekhem symbol is activated at the first attunement and is further energized and amplified at each of the six successive attunements so as to incrementally increase the empowerment and strength of this important and powerful symbol. This procedure also gradually introduces and furthers the process of unifying the Heaven and Earth aspects of Seichim and Reiki into the SSR trinity. When I asked my guides for information on the symbol's specific uses, I was enthusiastically told, "APPLY LIBERALLY."

The infinity symbol is the figure eight and in numerology has several meanings, including being the number of the Christ Consciousness and of resurrection and ascension. In *Jesus Christ, Sun of God*, David Fideler writes that the triple-eight number of "888" is "the number of Jesus" which is "a perfect name encompassing the whole of creation... ." Upright the figure eight represents the universal law of "As above, so below" as well as the balance between the spiritual and material worlds. Heaven and Earth also come together as one in the figure eight.

Infinity is limitless and without beginning or end. The energy of all polarities flows in both directions through the circles, meeting in the center of the figure eight at the unity or void point. This point of intersection is a portal or gateway to higher knowledge. The infinity pattern may be used to help balance the flow of energy in all areas of the physical and subtle bodies including the chakras. The infinity symbol can also be used to balance the flow between a person and his or her relationships with other people as well as with the situations or circumstances of life (such as how he or she relates to abundance or success).

As a person attains a state of higher consciousness, the two sides of the infinity pattern return to total and complete unification, merging into one central figure or sun. The sun rising above the infinity symbol is the Great Central Sun and is the One Source of all universes and All That Is. Here is the great I Am Presence of the Creator. Here is the Source of ALL LOVE.

Draw the Central Sun portion of the Heart of the Christos by making a clockwise circle with either hand. It is not necessary to draw the eight rays coming off of the Central Sun unless guided to do so. Draw the infinity starting at the center point moving your hand first in a clockwise circle back to the center point and then around counterclockwise to complete the figure eight. You may draw the Sun first and then the infinity pattern, or draw them in reverse order. You may also use either the Central Sun or the infinity sign alone when so inspired.

Another application of Heart of the Christos provided by SSR Master Teacher, Lesley Stoune, is to invert it so that the infinity portion is on the top and the

SSR Symbols: Heart of Gaia, an alternative form of Heart of the Christos

sun portion is on the bottom which serves to further ground the energy within a person. In her words:

One day I was really flying high. I was very happy and energetic but not at all well grounded. I had been making a habit of blessing all my food and drink with Heart of the Christos before eating. I had poured a glass of soda and had my hands wrapped around the glass to bless it. I opened up to draw in the SSR energy and formed the Heart of the Christos symbol in my mind, but it came upside down! I tried to turn it right side up but it flipped right back around.... I was very bothered by this and more or less forced it to stay right side up long enough to bless the soda. But, somewhere in the back of my mind was the "knowing" that the symbol had been sent upside down to help ground me. This thought stayed with me so I began working with Heart of the Christos inverted to see how other people and I reacted....

I believe Heart of the Christos upright represents the connection from our heart upward to the divine and that Heart of the Christos inverted represents the part of our central light column that projects from the heart down into the Earth. For this reason, I have come to think of the inverted symbol as the Heart of Gaia or Heart of the Earth.

Lesley has taken her experience even one step further by bringing together both an upright and an inverted Heart of the Christos to form a symbol that she calls Divine Balance shown below. She describes Divine Balance as follows:

> Used together, as a symbol with a sun both above and below the infinity symbol, I have found it to be a powerful balancing tool—Divine Balance. In drawing this symbol, I found that the serpentine movements connecting the "suns" with the infinity symbol created a beautiful curling symbol all its own.

Because Divine Balance is an extension of Heart of the Christos, it is not necessary to have an attunement specifically for this symbol in order to use it. To draw Divine Balance, begin with the sun that is above the infinity symbol by moving your hand in a clockwise motion as per arrow 1. At the point where the circle of the sun is completed, curve your hand down to the center of where the infinity symbol will be. Draw the infin-

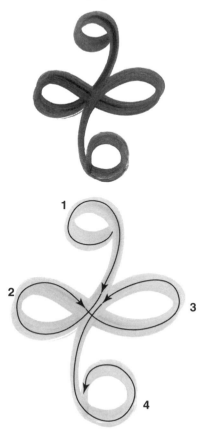

SSR Symbols: Divine Balance

ity symbol by going from the center to the left clockwise (arrow 2) and then complete the other half of the infinity going counterclockwise (arrow 3) and come back to the center point. From here, follow the downward curling of arrow 4 and draw the sun in the lower portion in a counterclockwise motion.

Integrating and Working with the Sekhem-Seichim-Reiki Sacred Symbols

When you begin using the SSR symbols after an attunement by an SSR Master Teacher, there is a period of time during which the symbols are being integrated into your energy structure. This takes place naturally following an attunement as a person adjusts to the new frequencies as well as when he or she is working with others during sessions. The length of this period varies from person to person and can be as short as a few weeks or months and as long as one or more years. Sometimes one of the symbols may be integrated very quickly and easily by an individual while another may take much longer.

There is no single factor that is determinative of the length of time for integration as the SSR energy meets a person where he or she is and then moves the person forward from there. The clearer a person is from an energetic perspective, the greater the likelihood of faster integration and grounding of the higher light frequencies invoked by a given symbol. Thus, doing your own personal healing work will greatly advance this process. In addition, there are several other methods you can use to help ground the symbols within your being:

- Practice drawing and writing the name of each symbol on paper and say its name aloud three times. Do this over and over.

- Meditate on each symbol one at a time while in a state of acceptance and simply observe each symbol's energy frequencies.

- Gaze at a symbol for a few minutes. Then close

your eyes and place the symbol on the screen of your third eye. Chant the name of the symbol over and over while looking at it on the inner screen. Should the image of the symbol fade or be difficult to perceive, open your eyes, gaze at the symbol again for a few moments, then close your eyes and begin chanting its name once more. As the third eye opens, you will eventually be able to hold the picture of the symbol on the inner screen.

In the early stages of learning to use a given SSR symbol during a client session, sign it once and say its name silently three times. It is important when actually drawing a symbol to follow the order and directional pattern indicated by the numbers and arrows. At first, use large movements whenever possible, as this will stimulate the learning pathways within the brain and trigger a deeper process of integrating the symbol. After practicing in this manner for a period of time, the learning becomes so profound that you will be able to make full connection with the symbol even when drawing it very small.

Eventually you will be able to visualize and project each symbol with full power from the third eye or by beaming it from your hands while saying the name of the symbol only once. You may well reach a point where you have so totally integrated a symbol that your higher self automatically conveys its power whenever needed, making it redundant and unnecessary to formally invoke the symbol during a session. This latter stage requires that you be a clear channel and may take some time to actualize.

Another way to ground the SSR symbols is to work with them as a grouping rather than individually by using what Phoenix Summerfield called a "string of beads" (a string of beads is also sometimes called a "string of jewels"). Take each of the symbols you have been attuned to in the order you received them and string them together in a row. Work with the resulting string of beads as a grouping to incorporate and maximize all of the learning you have received into a synthesized whole using the same methods described above.

In SSR, the order in which the SSR symbols are usually taught is: Cho Ku Rei "A," Cho Ku Rei "B," Sei He Ki, Hon Sha Ze Sho Nen, Reiki Dai Ko Myo, Seichim Dai Ko Myo, Cho Ku Ret, Shining Everlasting Flower of Enlightenment, Shining Everlasting Living Waters of Ra, Shining Everlasting Living Facets of Eternal Compassionate Wisdom and Healing and Heart of the Christos (Heart of the Christos is attuned at all seven facets). Therefore, this listing is the string of beads for the entire SSR system. However, if you have not been attuned to all of the SSR facets (see the section entitled Teaching Sekhem-Seichim-Reiki on page 96), you will not have received all 11 SSR symbols. Your string of beads would consist of those symbols that you have received with Heart of the Christos being the last symbol in the string of beads. If, for example, you have been attuned through the fourth facet of SSR, your string of beads would begin with Cho Ku Rei "A," go through Cho Ku Ret and then end with Heart of the Christos. See the two String of Beads charts in the section entitled Sekhem-Seichim-Reiki Practitioner and Master Teacher Attunements beginning on page 99.

As you work more closely with the SSR symbols, your understanding and integration of each one will continually deepen and evolve over time. You can facilitate this ongoing process by opening to the universal consciousness inherent in each symbol while asking to be imbued with the greater knowledge and wisdom of your higher self, which already knows the true meaning of the symbols. As you continue to evolve and integrate higher light frequencies, so too will your understanding of SSR and its related symbols unfold into infinity.

Symbols from Other Seichim Systems

In addition to the SSR symbols, there are several other symbols that have come to be associated with some of the many Seichim healing systems available today. From the beginning, many of those who have become involved with some form of Seichim have received more symbols while channeling, in dreams or through another person or teacher. Often they are guided to integrate these new symbols into their work with whatever system they are using and teaching, like I did with SSR. Because the energy stream is infinite, this is not surprising. The beauty of this process is that as one person grounds a facet of the SKHM universal diamond in symbolic form and shares it with another, this automatically makes the frequencies associated with the symbol accessible to everyone.

This phenomenon underscores the fact that although Dr. Usui and Patrick Zeigler are credited with bringing Reiki and Seichim/SKHM, respectively, to the modern world, the process has been, is, and will continue to be a collaborative adventure. This significant undertaking requires us to learn to work and share together in the true spirit of harmony, cooperation, partnership and unity. Though there are numerous symbols and systems available today, ultimately, like us, they are all One and the same and come from the Source of ALL LOVE.

Though it is not within the scope of this Guidebook to discuss these other Seichim symbols in detail, they are provided in the following sections with brief explanations in order to give the reader a greater appreciation of the wide variety of Seichim symbols that are in use today. I have included only those that are not already a part of SSR.

Isis Seichim

A Seichim system that originated in Australia for which I have received attunements as a Master Teacher is known as Isis Seichim. Isis Seichim is one of several Seichim systems that sprang up in Australia after Phoenix Summerfield began teaching there. These systems include New Life Seichim (Margot Deepa Slater), Sekhem (Helen Belot) and Seichim/Sekhem (Mary Shaw). Though there is some variation in the content and form of these systems, all of them have Phoenix's teachings as their foundation.

The information I have about Isis Seichim, its lineage and the symbols associated with it comes from the Isis Seichim manual provided to me by my teacher, Natalie Barton. Information about the lineage and symbols was also gleaned from an early Seichim manual written by Margot Deepa Slater that she provided to her first Seichim teacher, Marsha Nityankari Burack, in the months following her original attunements, as well as from a Seichim/Sekhem manual written by Stephen Comee. Patrick Zeigler and Nityankari also provided more pieces of the puzzle.

From what I have been able to gather, Isis Seichim was introduced by Ruth Mays (and possibly Mary Shaw per Stephen Comee's manual). The combined Reiki and Seichim lineage shown in my Isis Seichim manual is:

- Mikao Usui [Reiki]
- Chujiro Hayashi
- Hawayo Takata
- Arthur Robertson
- Ruth Mays [addition of Seichim to Reiki lineage]
- Inga Crisp
- Barbara Hedger
- Natalie Barton

What this family tree does not mention is Mary Shaw's possible involvement. It also does not take the Australian branch of the Seichim tree backward through Helen Belot (Mary and possibly Ruth's teacher), Margot Deepa Slater (Helen's original teacher), Marsha Nityankari Burack (Deepa's original teacher in the United States) and Phoenix Summerfield (Deepa, Helen and Nityankari's second teacher). From Phoenix, the tree goes back even further (see the section on the Seichim/SKHM history, on page 13, and Appendices III and IV for Phoenix's background).

I was unable to trace certain of the Isis Seichim symbols shown in the illustrations to Phoenix or any other Seichim teachers such as Tom Seaman. However, I found all of the ones in question in Margot Deepa Slater's early Seichim manual mentioned above. Therefore, since Deepa is one of the earliest if not the first person in Australia to be involved with Seichim, it is highly possible that she may have originated those that did not come from Phoenix. My efforts to locate Deepa to discuss this were unsuccessful.

Three of the symbols from Isis Seichim include a spiral or the infinity pattern and can be drawn to the power of three, seven or nine, where three "brings in the energy," seven "creates a deeper energy link" and nine "creates a total spiritual connection." These symbols include an alternate version of Cho Ku Rei, Ta Ku Rei and a symbol called Mai Yur Ma. In Isis Seichim, an alternative name for Mai Yur Ma is "Shining Everlasting Flower of Enlightenment" (recall that two other names used by Tom Seaman and Phoenix for the SSR symbol, Shining Everlasting Flower of Enlightenment, are "Mayooora" and "Mayourma").

These three symbols are depicted in the column to the right to the power of three. The powers of seven or nine can be accomplished by adding either four or six additional spirals or infinity patterns with each one being drawn slightly larger than the last.

Cho Ku Rei is called a magnifier that "empowers and magnifies all the other symbols, activating the property of making things whole." Ta Ku Rei is described as including the infinity pattern which "expands outwards to the infinite and finishes at the heart chakra." It is used for the same purposes as Cho Ku Rei with the choice of which one to use depending on the preference of the client. (Note Ta Ku Rei's similarity to Cho Ku Ret which was given to Patrick Zeigler by Marat. Note also T'om told me that he spells the name of this symbol as "Tankurhet.") Mai Yur Ma is characterized as "the gateway to the soul via the heart chakra ... which enhances, expands and magnifies the physical, emotional and spiritual aspects of unconditional love."

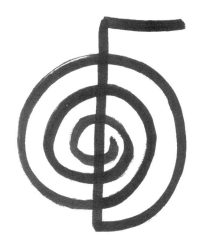

Isis Seichim Symbols: Cho Ku Rei (another version)

Isis Seichim Symbols: Ta Ku Rei

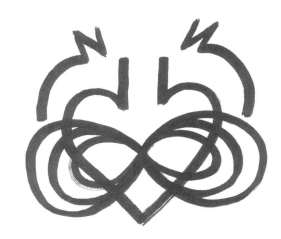

Isis Seichim Symbols: Mai Yur Ma

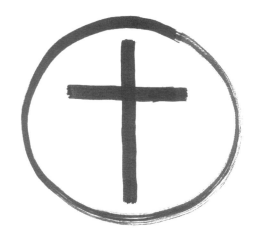

Isis Seichim Symbols: Symbol of Divinity

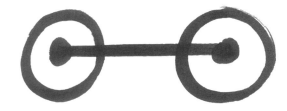

Isis Seichim Symbols: Merge Consciousness

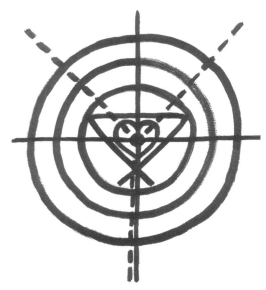

Isis Seichim Symbols: Eternal Pearl of Wisdom and Love

There are four other Isis Seichim symbols of interest. They are the Symbol of Divinity, Merge Consciousness, the Eternal Pearl of Wisdom and Love and the Healing Triangle and are shown to the left and below.

The Symbol of Divinity "directly addresses physical afflictions or problems caused by mental and emotional stress" and is a symbol of forgiveness and atonement. It also helps to "release the expectations of 'shoulds' and 'should nots'." For people of faiths other than Christianity, symbols such as the Om (Hinduism), Star of David (Judaism) and the Star and Crescent (Islam) may be substituted.

The Merge Consciousness symbol is used to "merge your consciousness with that of another person, animal, tree or plant." Eternal Pearl of Wisdom reflects the "eternal purity of the soul" and is the "gateway to destiny." Its vibrations move inward toward the heart. It is associated with the feminine and the qualities of purity, unity, truth, clarity, oneness, knowledge and wisdom. The Healing Triangle is used to "create a better situation or heal a problem at some level of the psyche." In Isis Seichim, the Healing Triangle is included as a symbol that is passed to a person through an attunement. Phoenix's Seichim system that I originally received refers to the healing triangle as a supplementary healing technique. Tom Seaman also remembers teaching students a similar method.

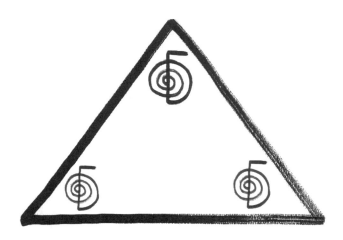

Isis Seichim Symbols: Healing Triangle

Additional Seichim Symbols

There are many other Seichim symbols that are in use today. Those included here are named Male-Female Balance, Eeef Tchay (sometimes spelled "Eeef Tchey"), Shum, Angel Wings, Align with God, Seichim Tao and yet another version of Shining Everlasting Flower of Enlightenment. They are depicted below and on the next page.

Male-Female Balance assists with bringing the masculine and feminine energies within a person into balance so as to foster unity and wholeness. Eeef Tchay influences the third eye to open into "endless inner sight." It dispels all illusion so that a person can see the truth of how things really are. Shum opens greater access to the joy and bliss associated with the higher levels of consciousness and is silent. Angel Wings gently inspires the realization of a person's full potential. It also seals and protects.

Align with God merges and aligns a person's higher, lower and God selves so that they are in accord, thus encouraging the person's highest good. Seichim Tao is about infinity, expansion, growth and entering other dimensions. This version of Shining Everlasting Flower of Enlightenment sits on the heart. It assists the person in releasing all negative and competitive masculine and feminine qualities and in bringing the energy of unconditional love into the heart.

In the Seichim community, it seems to be generally assumed that many, if not all, of the above symbols were originated by Tom Seaman during the first few years he was teaching. Several have also stated their belief that Phoenix Summerfield had a hand in the creation of some of them as well, while she and T'om were working together. After showing these additional Seichim symbols to T'om when we met, he indicated the following to the best of his recollection and knowledge:

- **Male-Female Balance** was created together by both Phoenix and T'om. Originally, it was called Shining Flower of Enlightenment by her (with the addition of two Cho Ku Ret symbols) and Mayooora by T'om as previously detailed in the discussion of the SSR version of this symbol. This version of the symbol most closely resembles the way in which Mayooora was drawn by T'om.
- **Eeef Tchay** combines two symbols with what T'om referred to as a "connector" symbol. T'om said that these symbols are from another language that was given to him by a swami. **Shum** is yet another symbol from this language.
- T'om believes that **Angel Wings** and **Align with God** were originated during the period when he and one of his students, Ken Lowry, were working together and doing some channeling.
- T'om was not familiar with **Seichim Tao** or this particular version of **Shining Everlasting Flower of Enlightenment**. Light and Adonea, whose Seichim manual contains these symbols, and their teacher, Geri Lennon, also could not shed any light on the question of their origination.

Additional Seichim Symbols: Male-Female Balance

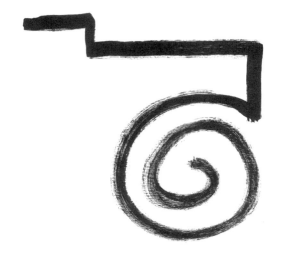

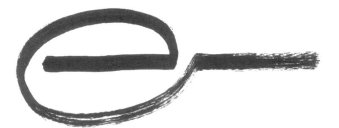

Additional Seichim Symbols: Shum

Additional Seichim Symbols: Eeef Tchay

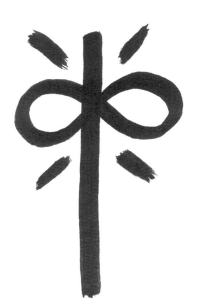

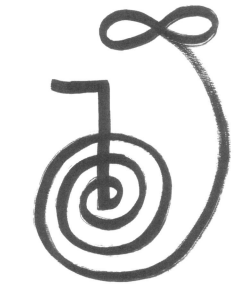

Additional Seichim Symbols: Seichim Tao

Additional Seichim Symbols: Align with God

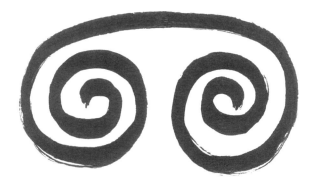

Additional Seichim Symbols: Angel Wings

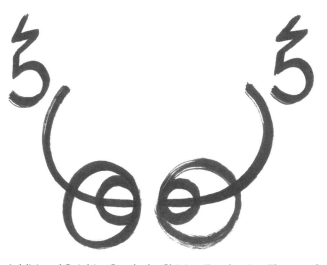

Additional Seichim Symbols: Shining Everlasting Flower of Enlightenment (another version)

Elements of an Energy Session

The many aspects of an SSR energy session are described below. Included are those elements that I have incorporated into my healing and counseling practice as a result of my personal experience, background, guidance and training as a licensed psychotherapist. The information is provided to give you a basic framework for a typical energy session as well as to demonstrate how you can integrate other disciplines and methods into a session to further develop your healing talents and assist those in need.

It is important to note that SSR and SKHM, by themselves, do not currently include the professional counseling skills and practices that are discussed primarily in the sections entitled Creating a Safe Emotional Space and Open Communication During a Session on pages 62 and 63. Most states require formal training and licensing before a healer can provide professional counseling to clients. For those readers who are licensed and trained to provide therapeutic consultations, I have provided this information to assist you in integrating SSR and SKHM into your therapeutic practices. If you are interested in becoming a professional therapist, check with the applicable universities, professional associations and state agencies for information.

Those elements of an energy session described below that do not involve professional counseling apply to all practitioners of SSR. After learning the basics and gaining some experience in working with the SSR and SKHM energy stream as discussed in this Guidebook, you are encouraged to bring your own uniqueness and background to you healing work, and to evolve it according to your own style, preferences, training and guidance.

Preparing the Physical Space

It is highly desirable to provide a safe, quiet, private and comfortable environment where the session will not be interrupted by outside distractions such as other people, pets, television, radio and the telephone. Have a blanket, pillow and tissues available. Play soft music in the background and light candles if desired. You also may wish to design the space according to Feng Shui principles to maximize the flow of the chi energy within the healing environment.

Set up the area where you will be seeing people to provide for your personal comfort as well. For example, an excellent investment that is greatly beneficial is a professional massage table that allows you to set the height according to your size so as to prevent strain on your body. It is also useful to have a chair and a pillow available in case you wish to sit down or kneel on the floor during the session.

It is good spiritual hygiene to energetically cleanse the room where sessions are given both before and after. Many space clearing methods are available for this purpose such as the use of essential oils and burning incense or sage. You can also use angelic light weaving (see page 72) or specifically call on your guides, angels, the ascended masters and the Source of ALL LOVE to clear the space. You may wish to use some form of sound, such as playing mantras or music or toning for a period of time. Another way to clear the space is to invoke and place the SSR symbols in the center of the room and on the walls, ceiling and floor. The SKHM Shenu also can be used for this purpose.

One of the most effective space clearing methods I know is the use of a fire pot. Find a deep pan that is no longer needed for cooking and place it on the floor in the middle of the room to be cleared. Put three to four tablespoons of Epsom salts in the pan. Pour in enough rubbing alcohol to fully wet and cover the salts.

Make sure to take the necessary fire precautions, such as placing something under the pan to protect whatever it is sitting on and avoiding burning the fire too close to papers, fabrics, furniture or hair.

Light the alcohol using a match and immediately stand back. The fire will burn for a few minutes and clear away negative mental, astral and emotional energies in the room and in the auric fields of the people in the room. Clean the residue left in the pan by soaking in warm water. An excellent book with more ideas about space clearing and that covers the basics of Feng Shui is *Sacred Space* by Denise Linn.

Preparing Yourself

Regular spiritual practices such as breathwork, contemplation, prayer, meditation and working with sound are excellent ways to ready yourself for a session. An internal focus that honors the session and the highest good of both the receiver and you is important. Clear the body, mind and emotions of distractions before beginning to allow divine guidance to enter and lead the healing work. Drink plenty of water before, during and after a session since water is an excellent energy conduit. Drinking water also helps to flush toxins out of the body.

Sometimes it is helpful in clearing toxins to take a cleansing bath before and/or after a session using sea salt, Epsom salts, baking soda or peroxide (the peroxide is highly diluted so it will not cause bleaching of the hair). You can also place a few drops of a favorite essential oil in the bath water. When the bath is complete, take a shower as normal. After drying off, place moisturizing lotion on the body. If you can only take a shower, an alternative is to make a paste of the sea salt, Epsom salts or baking soda and rub the paste on the body, including the chakra areas. When rinsing, request through clear intention that the shower clear the auric field as well.

It is also suggested that you wash your hands before and after an energy session. Besides obvious hygienic considerations, this ensures that there will be no undesirable energy transfer from one person to another. Washing also helps to clear and stop the energy flow in the hands. If water is not available, another method for stopping the energy flow is to place the hands against a wall or other flat surface for a few moments.

Creating a Safe Emotional Space

An essential part of supporting another person in his or her healing process is creating a safe emotional space. A safe emotional space is one in which both client and practitioner are able to be loving and respectful of one another in order to build trust and confidence in the relationship. This includes establishing a non-judgmental atmosphere in which effective listening and communication skills are practiced. Without this foundation, neither person will feel the security necessary to honestly share his or her true feelings and experience, which is central to being able to cultivate genuine healing.

In order to offer a safe space to others, a practitioner must learn to be safe within him or herself. If you have not healed and learned to feel comfortable with an issue within yourself such as death, anger or abuse, this will be silently communicated to your client, adversely affecting the comfort and trust level of the recipient. These unhealed areas of your life can also influence in an undesirable way your ability to effectively facilitate a person through such issues.

In the section entitled Qualities and Values of a Healing Practitioner and Teacher, beginning on pabe 82, I emphasize that the most essential quality is to be actively committed to your own healing process, including healing the shadow self and learning to take personal responsibility for all that happens in your life. The same section also discusses additional qualities to cultivate within yourself that will have a beneficial effect on your ability to offer a safe emotional space to others. Preparing the physical space and yourself as described above will also greatly enhance your efforts in this regard.

Another key to creating an atmosphere of safety and trust is recognizing that most often, it is not necessary for a client to relive the full extent of the emotions and pain associated with traumatic and painful experiences such as abuse. Many times the release can be accomplished gently, with either no pain at all or only a small proportion of the pain coming into the client's awareness. This is often enough to provide him or her with an understanding of what took place for the purpose of learning the applicable soul lesson. This is a blessing of grace and compassion given to us freely by the Source of ALL LOVE.

The art of right timing and readiness on the client's part for release of old programming and trauma is one that requires patience, understanding and compassion. Do not force or push. When I become aware that a client is swimming in potentially rough waters, I softly reassure and encourage him or her to continue. I also remind the person that he or she has the right to stop whatever we are doing at any time if the process becomes too frightening or uncomfortable. If the client indicates a desire to stop, I will gently ask a question or two as guided to see if it is possible for the client to keep going.

Often at this point all the client needs is some reassurance that he or she is safe and a reminder that your purpose in being present is to help support him or her to go through whatever is coming up with a minimum of pain. Sometimes the part of the client that wants to stop simply needs permission to feel exactly what it is feeling. However, if the client repeats that he or she wants to stop, I respect that request.

A safe emotional space is also fostered when both the recipient and the practitioner are fully clothed. It is usually desirable, however, to ask the person to remove a tight belt, shoes, watch, other jewelry and glasses to allow for maximum flow of the energy stream during the session. It is also wise and respectful to ask permission before physically touching an individual or working within his or her energy field. Take special care to touch the person in an appropri-

ate and professional manner, with particular sensitivity to those who may have experienced physical and/or sexual abuse and a lack of healthy personal boundaries.

Treat each individual with respect and honor his or her body temple. This, in turn, models healthy boundaries to the person. For some, this may be the first experience of feeling loving energy and true intimacy without any sexual connotation or other inappropriate violation of boundaries, which is a true learning and healing experience for all.

Length of a Session

Staying reasonably within the agreed time frame is also an important part of creating a safe space and learning about healthy boundaries for both the client and the practitioner. A session can be any length of time, usually between one and two hours. While a session may occasionally run longer for good reason, take care to maintain an overall energetic balance and flow of giving and receiving that honors both the recipient's and the practitioner's needs.

This is an important lesson, since those in the helping professions often have the tendency to overextend themselves, which ultimately serves no one and can lead to burnout. When the practitioner treats him or herself with respect by honoring the agreed-to time boundaries, he or she will similarly be communicating a healthy and balanced perspective to the client.

Open Communication During a Session

Some kind of open verbal exchange is very useful at the beginning of the session. The practitioner can learn more about the person and why he or she has come for assistance, or the two can share what the person has experienced since his or her previous session. When I meet with a client for the first time, we discuss the person's situation as well as his or her desired goals.

This is also a good time to explain how the session will flow, including answering questions the client may have about SSR and how you approach the healing process. This is especially important when the person has had little or no previous energy work of a similar nature. The discussion allows the person to clear his or her mind early on in the session. I also like to make sure the person has at least a general appreciation of the human energy system.

I explain to the person some of the body sensations that he or she may feel during the session, such as tingling, temperature changes, shifts in the breathing rhythm, lightheadedness and vibration. I describe some of the common experiences he or she might have such as feelings of overall relaxation, peace, joy and love as well as the release of emotions such as anger and sadness, along with the need to cry. I explain that the client may also remember experiences from this or other lifetimes that are ready to be cleared.

After completing the above discussion, and before proceeding with the energy work portion of the session, you may wish to have your client sign a consent form which discloses pertinent information in writing to the person about SSR and the healing process. You will also want to be sure to document the session in writing. For a full discussion of these topics, see the section entitled Professional Standards of Care, on page 86, as well as Appendix VIII, on page 133, for a Sample SSR Client Consent Form and Appendix IX, on page 137, for a Sample SSR Client Summary Form.

After you have begun the actual energy work, additional conversation and questioning may take place during portions of the session, while in others there may be complete silence. The rhythm of this ebb and flow will vary between clients and with each session. Knowing when to be silent and learning to be comfortable within the seemingly "empty" space is important. Much can be taking place inside the person that requires his or her complete inner attention.

The facilitating questions I ask during a session are geared toward assisting the client to find his or her own answers. Though I may already intuitively sense what is going on within the person, it is always more empowering for the client to discover this for him or herself. This also teaches the client how to do search for his or her own answers and furthers the process of the person taking responsibility for the healing process. In deciding what questions to ask, I simply follow the flow of the energy of the person through observation and intuitive guidance.

For example, while working on the person's heart chakra, you may be inspired to ask the question, "What does forgiveness mean to you?" The client answers. You then follow up by asking, "Is there some situation in your life or some person—even yourself—where forgiveness might be needed?" The client answers again, and you continue the exchange based on where the client's energy leads you, while also using the various healing tools you have available such as the SSR symbols, angelic light weaving and toning (see the sections on these topics for more information).

When questioning a client during a session, I follow the general guideline of inviting the person to delve more deeply into a given issue no more than three times. I adopted this rule of thumb from the work of Elisabeth Kubler-Ross, a psychiatrist most well known for her work in the field of death and dying. I saw a video of hers years ago in which she discussed her approach to emotional healing. She stated that to go beyond three attempts in encouraging a client is to impose your own will. It is always the client's choice as to how far to go with the process.

This has always felt like sage advice, especially since I have both observed and been on the receiving end of well-intended, yet misguided healers who by their insistent pushing have reinforced the trauma rather than healing it. The art of the healing work you do is helping to support a person in gently stretching beyond his or her usual boundaries while not being too forceful or trying to go too fast. If you cross over this line, you risk eroding the trust and sense of safety you have established. This can also provoke enough of a fear response in the client that he or she shuts down and becomes unwilling to venture again into the same territory for quite some time to come.

You may receive guidance saying that it is appropriate to share with the recipient particular information your spirit guides or angels have given to you. It is wise to ask the person if he or she would like to hear the information. If the answer is yes, relay the details without judgment in a compassionate and loving way. Give the person the choice to either accept or reject the information as relevant to his or her life. Do not impose the guidance you receive about a client as absolute truth. It is also best to report channeled material exactly as received without interpretation. Many times a phrase, word, image or name that has no meaning to you means everything to the other person.

Opening Prayer or Invocation

Some form of opening prayer or invocation is helpful because it is part of setting the intention and evoking the energy for the session. The prayer or invocation may be said silently or aloud. My preference is to say the prayer out loud so that the recipient is included, although I must admit to feeling very self-conscious about doing this in my early years of being a practitioner.

I use a modified version of the soul mantra originally channeled by Alice Bailey because of its power and its ability to quicken the healing and ascension process. It is also a beautiful complement to SSR. The modified mantra is as follows:

I am the Soul.

I am the Monad.

I am the Light Divine.

I am Love.

I am Will.

I am Perfect Design.

This mantra opens the central light channel and the chakras and invokes all planes of existence to assist in the healing session. Recite the mantra three

times at the very beginning of the session going through the entire verse before repeating it again. I usually substitute "We Are . . . " for "I Am ... " when working with a client so that both of us are included in the invocation. Another way to use the mantra is to recite each line, and then ask the client to repeat it.

This ancient mantra was given to the world some years ago by an ascended master named Djwhal Khul through Alice Bailey. According to her writings (see the Bibliography), no work of a spiritual nature should be undertaken until this mantra or some form of it has been said. Otherwise, all meditations, chanting, healing techniques and similar efforts will be ineffective in making lasting changes in the physical and subtle bodies.

Repetition of the first two lines brings about identification with the soul and the monad. The next four lines are spoken "as if" the person is the soul and monad to assist the human personality in learning to identify first with the soul and then with the monad. As this process continues, the personality will cooperate with the soul and monad more frequently, and the building of a person's central light column and light body will be further stimulated.

I am the Soul. When you say this invocation of the soul, the statement activates the spark of the soul star, which is six inches above the head. The radiance of the soul star intensifies and may extend several feet. The soul star is not the soul. Rather, it is the etheric symbol of that portion of the soul that is linked with matter and is the instrument through which the soul does its work. "I am the Soul" is another way of saying, "I am the Christ Consciousness."

I am the Monad. After you have identified with the soul or Christ Consciousness, this statement aligns the soul and the incarnated personality with its monad. Each of the infinite number of monads is made up of groups or families of many individual spiritual sparks of the Creator. The monad is at the level of the I Am Presence. This statement is not part of the mantra channeled by Alice Bailey. I have added it because, according to Joshua David Stone's writings, it invokes identification at the next level beyond the soul, which many people today are ready to do. See Chapter 16 of his book, *Cosmic Ascension,* for his explanation of the nine levels of the soul mantra.

I am the Light Divine. As this line is recited, the central light column flashes as it becomes full of rainbow fire. This activates and moves a person into the level of the higher abstract mind.

I am Love. With this invocation, the central channel floods with a rose pink downpour of energy from the heart of the soul star. The recipient enters into the buddhic plane, the plane of pure love, pure reason, intuitional knowing and total Oneness with the Christ Consciousness and the I Am Presence.

I am Will. A downpour of some combination of royal purple, brilliant clear red, white and indigo blue light enters and fills the central channel as the line is recited. This downpour is the atmic principle, i.e., the realization of self as spiritual will.

I am Perfect Design. This statement causes the chakras along the central light column to flash and intensify. "Perfect design" refers to the plan or blueprint of the soul for the current incarnation. This statement is the acknowledgment of one's soul purpose in its purest and highest form. "I am Perfect Design" was originally channeled by Alice Bailey as "I am Fixed Design."

Because the wording of this mantra may be unfamiliar to some, I usually explain when a person comes for the first session that I will be using an opening prayer that his or her conscious mind may not fully comprehend. I assure the recipient that on a soul level, he or she does know the meaning of the prayer and that later on I will be happy to answer all questions about it. I find this helps to keep the client's mental body from distracting him or her from the experience of the session.

Light Helpers

Your next step in a session is invoking the assistance of the I Am Presence—the Source of ALL LOVE—and the higher self and spirit guides of both the client and you. Also call on those guides, angels, archangels, teachers and ascended masters of the highest levels of clear light who are available to assist with the session. Although my preference is to do this aloud, it may also be done in silence. All beings called upon are intended to be present for the highest good. Include prayers of gratitude and acknowledgment for their healing presence and help.

If there is a specific presence for whom you are guided to ask, call on that light being by name. If you do not know the specific name, invoke the presence by function or characteristic, for example, the archangel of healing or the archangel of forgiveness. Also ask the recipient to bring in any additional light beings he or she wishes to have participate in the session by naming them aloud or in the silence of his or her heart. I prefer to have the client do this aloud because it gives me a good indication of how well the person understands and relates to the ascended realms. The following invocation is the type I use most often:

> *Mother Goddess/Father God, I Am Presence and the Source of ALL LOVE: We come before you and ask for the presence of those healing guides, masters, teachers and angels of the highest levels of the clear light to be here now to participate in this healing session. Specifically, we ask for the presence of _____ (fill in the names of those specific light beings you wish to have present, such as Archangel Michael, Jesus, Mother Mary, Quan Yin or others based on your intuitive sense of whom to ask. Then invite the client to call in any others whom he or she wishes to be present).*

There are many levels of assistance available including the Egyptian gods and goddesses; the gods and goddesses of all other traditions such as Atlantian, Hindu, Buddhist, Hawaiian and Native American; the saints and ascended masters; the archangels and angels; and the many councils within the higher light dimensions and their associated evolved light beings. One may also call directly on the Source of ALL LOVE. Since the physical body is made up of the elements of the Earth, remember to call on Mother Earth and her spirits for healing assistance, including the elemental devas, fairies and gnomes. Earth energy is also useful to call on when a client is not well grounded in his or her body.

Consciously invoking the assistance of the many ascended light beings and the Source of ALL LOVE greatly enhances the entire healing process. Though these light beings and the Source of ALL LOVE are already everywhere at once, the universal law of free will says they cannot intervene in someone's life except upon invitation or when the person's life is in danger before his or her time. Making it clear that you consciously desire and welcome their presence and assistance allows their grace and compassion to more fully enter your life and helps to build and strengthen your connection with them.

Sometimes a particular ascended master may come in very strongly and wish for you to make his or her presence known to the client, which can be especially meaningful to the person. Your modeling of the process of calling on the ascended realms for guidance and support also helps the client to open to and establish his or her own connection with these loving and compassionate beings and the Source of ALL LOVE.

Even if you are unable to fully witness the presence of these beautiful beings through your inner senses, i.e., clairvoyance (inner seeing), clairsentience (inner feeling), claircognizance (inner knowing), and clairaudience (inner hearing), learn to trust and have confidence that they are with you. As you cultivate higher levels of trust and acceptance within yourself, your facility in working with the higher realms will likewise increase.

For years I have used a formula in learning to develop my ability to work with guidance from the higher realms: ALAA. This acronym stands for ASK, LISTEN, ACCEPT and ACT. Ask for guidance. Be open and sensitive to and listen for the many ways guidance will come to you during sessions. Learn to accept and trust the guidance without questioning, doubting or negating it. The last step is to take positive action based on the guidance.

Your faith in the intuitive wisdom you receive will grow into a full appreciation of the assistance available on many levels. Remembering that all of us are a part of the Source of ALL LOVE's light and wisdom in each and every moment allows the perfect answers to be brought forth. An excellent book to help you develop your skills in this area is *Divine Guidance* by Doreen Virtue, Ph.D.

Healing Intention and Prayer

At this point, I usually ask the recipient to take a moment to tune into the consciousness of his or her heart and allow the heart to share what the person's healing needs are at that moment. Often I place one of my hands on or above the heart chakra to enhance the person's ability to access the wisdom of the heart. I then request that the client say aloud the heart's answer in the form of a healing intention and prayer that expresses what he or she wishes to receive and heal.

The healing intention and prayer serves several purposes, including helping the person define what he or she truly needs and wants. It also empowers the individual to create this result and strongly encourages him or her to take active responsibility for the healing process. Conceiving and then saying the healing intention aloud from the heart is an active process that increases the probability of its manifestation beyond mere thought and desire.

Saying the intention aloud also increases the likelihood of the person being willing to take the actions required to make those changes in his or her life that would support the healing process. Speaking the answer helps open the throat chakra and connect it to the heart so that the words spoken reflect the individual's genuine truth and deepest heart's desires. Though the possibilities are endless, some examples of a healing request might be:

- I want to heal my relationship with my parents.
- I want to understand the lessons involving my illness.
- I want to let go of the pattern that keeps attracting emotionally unavailable men/women to me (or any other pattern).
- I want to experience joy and deal with those things that have caused me to be so sad.
- I want to enhance communication with my spirit guides and angels.
- I want a loving, caring and committed relationship with a man/woman.
- I want to expand and further open my heart chakra (or any others that may need work).
- I want to deal with and release the anger (sadness, grief, worry, etc.) and have more peace in my life.
- I want to know my life's purpose and the steps I need to take to bring it to fruition this lifetime.

Encourage the person to come from his or her heart and to be thoughtful and thorough, taking whatever time is needed to formulate the healing intention and prayer. There is no limit to what can be asked for and actualized. If the prayer is too general or vague, i.e., "I want to heal myself," gently prompt the person to be more specific by asking a question such as, "What within yourself would you like to heal?" Listen carefully to what is said and how it is said. It will give you important direct and intuitive information and clues about areas within the recipient's energy system that may need attention during the session.

It has been my experience that some kind of answer to the person's healing request invariably comes during the session. For instance, a client may want to clear a pattern dealing with his or her mother. As an example of what could happen, you may find yourself intuitively drawn to place your hands on the solar plexus region. As you offer energy to this area, the client may begin to remember an event he or she has not thought of for years and begin to cry. A past life memory might also surface as you continue to provide gentle support, encouragement and additional SSR energy. As these memories are shared, you might find yourself guided to help the client in releasing the associated feelings and thoughts.

Therefore, I regard whatever happens during a session as some form of direct response to the person's healing request. I do my best to observe these responses and then, if need be, assist the client in becoming conscious of the ways in which the answer has been received. This helps the client to become more aware of the powerful effect his or her words and intention have on the healing process.

Opening the Central Light Column with the Breath

After completing the healing request, I guide the person through the following simple breathing process to gently and gradually open and expand the central column as well as ground him or her to the Source of ALL LOVE and the heart of the Earth. The process will also help open any blocked or congested energy pathways to release suppressed negative patterning from the cellular memory and reprogram the cells with healing light and love. Everything is gradually dissolved that stands in the way of the nourishing and natural circulation of blood, oxygen and light energy within the physical, emotional, mental and spiritual bodies.

Take care to allow adequate time between each phase for the person to complete the instruction. Also, since many people are not visually oriented, assure the person that he or she does not have to actually "see" the column and everything that is happening during the opening. The intention to complete the meditation is all that is required. The steps for breathing open the column are as follows:

1. Ask the person to breathe more deeply and slowly than normal, breathing in up from the lungs through the shoulders and to the top of the head, then breathing out all the way down to the bottom of the feet. Suggest that the individual do this several times, creating a circular flow of energy around the entire body. Encourage the inhalation and exhalation to be even in length.

2. After the person has begun to relax and quiet down, suggest that he or she become aware of the central light column that runs vertically through the middle of the body from the top of the head to the bottom of the feet, parallel to the spine and connecting the chakras. (If the person is seated, his or her awareness should be brought to the column running vertically from the top of the head to the base of the spine.) Ask the person to then open and expand the column by gently breathing in and out several times.

3. Next ask the person to picture his or her feet standing firmly on the Earth and to send the column down like roots from a tree all the way into the center or heart of the Earth and then to anchor it there.

4. Now ask the person to also extend the column above the head all the way through the celestial realms up to the heart of the Source of ALL LOVE and anchor it there.

5. Ask the person to continue the same breathing rhythm, simultaneously breathing the grounding and supportive Earth energies into the column from below and the celestial Heaven energies into the column from above, allowing Heaven and Earth to come together within the heart region. Here the energies blend, merge, balance and unify as One and fill up the heart to capacity.

6. Encourage the person to permit the unified energies to then spill over into the entire circulatory system of the physical body, nourishing all the tissues, organs, muscles, bones and cells. Then have the person expand the flow from the heart like a

sunburst into the etheric, emotional, mental and spiritual bodies that surround and interpenetrate the physical body.

For the balance of the SSR session, healing energies that support and enhance the work will now be circulated through the central light column, into the heart, then on to the physical and subtle bodies as the person continues to inhale and exhale. Gently remind the person to reestablish the deeper and slower breathing rhythm whenever he or she lapses back into a shallow breathing pattern during the course of the session.

If so guided, you can also expand Step 6 above to gradually move the unified energies one step at a time into each of the subtle bodies using the breath and taking whatever time is needed at each level. This will allow the unified frequencies additional time to cleanse and purify the body and each of the auric field layers, offering the client a greater opportunity to fully absorb and integrate these frequencies into his or her total energy system. When approaching Step 6 in this expanded way, I sometimes am guided to offer the client some explanation, as I find this helps him or her to become more aware of what is happening at each of the levels.

An alternative method for opening the central column at this point in a healing session is to lead the recipient through the SKHM Group Attunement Meditation or do an SKHM Healing Attunement. These methods are discussed more fully in the section entitled Patrick Zeigler's Approach to Healing with SKHM, on page 26, and in Appendices V and VI.

Opening Spiral

At this point in the session, I use a clockwise opening spiral if so guided. You can use either your right or left hand for creating the spiral depending on your preference. This technique was taught to me by my first Reiki Master, John Harvey Gray. The spiral further opens the client's energy field for the session.

Begin by gently holding your hand palm down above the person's heart chakra for a moment. In a clockwise spiraling motion, sweep your hand next to the solar plexus, briefly pausing to hold your hand above this area. From the solar plexus, move in a clockwise spiraling motion to the throat chakra and hold for a moment. Continue moving from the throat to the sacral chakra, then to the third eye chakra, root chakra, crown chakra, Earth star—which is about six inches below the feet—and finally the soul star, which is about six inches above the top of the head. This completes the pattern of the opening spiral.

While you are completing the spiral, you can begin the process of scanning the person's chakras with your hand. As you sweep your hand across the body in the opening spiral, notice which chakras are open and moving, how much they are moving and in what direction. This provides valuable information on general areas of blockage that might need to be addressed during the session. See the next section for further information on scanning the body.

Scanning the Body

An important part of SSR is learning to scan the body and the chakras. This allows the practitioner to check the flow of the life force energy within all areas of the physical, emotional, mental and spiritual bodies. When scanning, take your time to feel the flow of energy in the aura around the body, which is continuously shifting according to the physical, emotional, mental and spiritual states of the person. You will notice these changes through your outer senses, including through your hands, which may register sensations such as tingling, prickling, heaviness, thickness or pressure. The energetic shifts can also be noted through the inner senses such as clairvoyance, clairsentience, clairaudience and claircognizance.

There is much information you may become aware of while scanning the physical and subtle bodies, such as temperature changes, directional and vibrational energy movement or lack thereof, colors and color changes within an area, sounds and varying tones being made by the body, the level of functioning of the chakras, distinctive odors, and the height and depth of an area, indicating when you are moving from one energy body to another. All of these are important sources of information regarding the general condition of the client's electromagnetic field.

When scanning, simply note your impressions and observations without judging them or deciding what they mean. Once you have finished scanning, go back and double-check the areas that were particularly noteworthy. Take into account that symptoms could be showing up in one or more of the subtle bodies as well as in the physical body. If you wish, you may discuss your impressions with the client and ask for feedback on possible symptoms or imbalances in those areas. This feedback is invaluable because it can help you confirm and fine-tune your observations. However, sometimes the client will not be able to supply you with any information about an area you mention. This does not necessarily invalidate your observation.

The following are general examples of scanning results. A hot or warm place on the body may be an area that is currently injured, inflamed, over-energized, highly stressed or diseased. It may also be suggestive of a chronic problem. On the other hand, coolness often indicates a block in the flow of energy to the area, including possible congestion within the circulatory system of the physical and subtle bodies. Coolness may also be an energy leak within the auric field. Blocks and congestion within a body system or an organ may show up as a thick or heavy feeling. Thickness and heaviness may further hint at a vulnerable area that requires additional protection.

For more information on understanding the results of a scan, you can refer to various models of the human energy system, such as are used in acupuncture, that show the correspondence of body systems, glands and organs to the chakras and meridians. Barbara Brennan's book, *Hands of Light*, is also an excellent reference in this regard.

ELEMENTS OF AN ENERGY SESSION

I believe that each practitioner and teacher must also develop over time his or her own unique energetic "reference library." This reference system grows out of the personal experience you gain while practicing energy work. In addition, your guides will take advantage of the ways in which you are already sensitive to the flow of their guidance. For example, I lean most naturally toward clairsentience and claircognizance, so much of the information I receive comes through in these ways. In the meantime, my other inner senses are also developing. Be assured that your guides will work with you to gradually develop all of your inner senses.

Learn to trust that you and your client will be provided whatever information is necessary for the client's highest good. Do not feel you have to be all-knowing or highly developed as a psychic in order to be an excellent practitioner and teacher.

Hand Positions

A basic traditional Reiki session usually involves treating areas on the front torso, as well as the head, neck, shoulders, arms, hands, legs and feet while a person is lying on his or her back. After the practitioner completes the front of the body, the person turns over and the head, neck, shoulders, back, lower torso, arms, hands, legs and feet are treated from the rear. The person then returns to lying on his or her back for completion of the session.

When working with Reiki energy by itself, the hands generally are lightly placed directly on the physical body following a prescribed series of hand positions. These positions are designed to include all of the key areas of the energetic system. Each position is held until the practitioner feels a rise and fall in the amount of energy being drawn, usually somewhere between three and five minutes. Please refer to the many available books on Reiki for a description of the most commonly used hand positions.

In contrast, the process is entirely intuitive and directed by Spirit when using the combined SSR energy matrix. As such, there is no "correct" set of hand positions nor a single prescribed protocol to follow when giving an SSR healing. You will energetically work both above and directly on the physical body using various techniques such as angelic light weaving, page 72, and sound healing, page 77.

Over time, you will learn to know and trust your intuition as it guides you through a session. Once again, nothing can replace the value of your accumulated practice and experience. Let small thoughts, feelings and messages that come to you during a session gently guide you in how you proceed, such as going to a particular place on the body and placing your hands there. Learn to trust a sense of being pulled or drawn toward an area of the body or the auric field. Feedback from the person receiving the healing is also a rich source of information to guide you during the session.

When a person reports any kind of condition present in the body, such as a headache, there is the temptation to go straight to the head, treat the symptom and not include other areas. While the course of the energy work will likely include working directly on the head, the source or cause of the problem is often somewhere else in one or more locations in the physical and subtle bodies, including the mental, emotional and spiritual bodies. Be thorough in your approach, going beyond the area where the "dis-ease" symptom is being experienced by the person. This applies to most, if not all, forms of major and minor symptoms.

The more you work with the energies of the SSR matrix, the stronger they will become within you and in your life. While touch is one of the main ways that SSR is activated, the energy stream becomes a part of your entire being, including your auric field, which allows you to consciously call on the SSR and SKHM energy stream through other means. Thus, SSR may also be activated through the eyes and as sound energy through the voice. It can be directed through your mind focus as thought. If you are an artist, singer, musician or writer, SSR can be channeled through your intention into your creative work. If you are speaking on the telephone, SSR energy can be transmitted to the other person through your voice and the intention of your thought.

Angelic Light Weaving

Angelic light weaving is a technique transmitted through the angelic kingdom that guides you in weaving the living light of the SSR energy stream in various patterns throughout a person's energy system. I learned the technique from a healer named Frank Alper and find that it beautifully complements and enhances the SSR energy matrix.

You may weave light above and below the receiver's entire body or weave it within a particular chakra or area of the body. The light weaving energies emanating from your hands and fingertips can be used as a form of aura cleansing as well as to assist the physical and various subtle bodies to realign, reintegrate and repattern. Imagine yourself as a mystical weaver, creating a cloth of light energy with clear, golden and other multicolored threads!

Angelic light weaving can be used at any time during a session to clear the physical space where you are working, scan the auric field, release undesirable energies and blocks and infuse a particular energetic quality into the auric field. The sacred symbols of the SSR energy matrix may also be woven into the auric field.

Call on the archangels and angels with your intention and invite their energetic flow to move through your heart chakra and into your arms and hands. Ask them to guide your arms and hands, as they are master light weavers. Relax yourself completely and allow your movements to be gentle, smooth and firm so as not to agitate the energy field.

One moment your hands may be above the person's head, where you feel drawn to light weave for a period of time. Next you may find yourself placing your hands directly on the feet for a few minutes, then beginning to light weave once again over the legs. From there you sense the need to place your hands on the person's shoulders for a time and so on. The creative possibilities for the various ways your hands and arms may move during angelic light weaving are endless.

Sometimes the motions of your light weaving will be large, and at other times tiny, intricate and delicate. The movements might be made in a pulling or scooping motion to draw out any energies being released from the physical and subtle bodies. You can also shoot SSR energy out the tips of your fingers like a laser beam to direct it to specific areas for cleansing and release. When used in this way, angelic light weaving can be thought of as a form of psychic surgery.

At certain times, you may be guided to light weave a particular vibrational energy for the benefit of the recipient such as forgiveness, courage or self-love. To accomplish this, you can call by name on the archangel or angel who oversees the desired quality. If you do not know the name, simply call on the energy stream of the quality itself, and this will bring forth the appropriate light being from the angelic realms to assist you with the light weaving. You also can simply ask to light weave whatever quality would be for the highest good of the client without having to specifically name it.

Angelic light weaving can be used in many other ways including enhancing vitamins or medicines, clearing stones and crystals, blessing food and sending healing energies to the Earth.

Using the Sekhem-Seichim-Reiki Sacred Symbols

IN GENERAL

An earlier section entitled The Sekhem-Seichim-Reiki Sacred Symbols, which begins on page 40, described the various purposes and applications of the symbols, including advice on how to learn and integrate them. All of the SSR symbols are available to support and empower the healing process. In some sessions, you may not use any of these symbols, while in others you may invoke numerous ones. Use intuitive guidance and your appreciation of the client's needs and desires to choose which symbols to invoke during a session

There is no better way to gain insight into the possible uses of a given symbol than invoking it and observing what takes place. Some effects may be easy to notice within the time frame of the session. Others may not be immediately apparent, yet over time the client may report feeling positive changes within him or herself. It is wise, therefore, to learn to trust when you are guided to use a particular symbol even if you are not able to connect all of the dots and see the whole healing picture at the time. Remember, the symbols work on very subtle levels and our understanding of their power and many applications is still unfolding.

INCREASING THE POWER LEVEL

There are three methods for increasing the amount of power being drawn by the practitioner for healing purposes during a session. One is invoking the symbol Cho Ku Rei "A." The second is known as a power sandwich. To invoke one, you would intuitively choose any of the SSR symbols to serve as the two pieces of "bread," then use your guidance to choose any combination of the 11 SSR symbols as the sandwich "filler."

You also may derive clues for choosing the appropriate "bread" symbol by considering the needs and goals of the client. For example, if the person desires to become aware of his or her soul purpose, it might be beneficial to use Shining Everlasting Flower of Enlightenment, which assists in discerning the soul's blueprint. Choose other symbols for the filler according to what intuitively feels appropriate. You can further amplify this power sandwich by placing two Cho Ku Rei "A"s on either side of the bread symbol. The symbols used in such a power sandwich follow with the actual symbols shown below:

- Cho Ku Rei "A"
- Shining Everlasting Flower of Enlightenment
- Hon Sha Ze Sho Nen
- Cho Ku Rei "B"
- Shining Everlasting Living Waters of Ra
- Reiki Dai Ko Myo
- Sei He Ki
- Cho Ku Ret
- Shining Everlasting Flower of Enlightenment
- Cho Ku Rei "A"

The third method for increasing power to its fullest is the use of a "string of beads" as described in the section entitled The Sekhem-Seichim-Reiki Sacred Symbols on page 54. You would draw on the combination of all of the SSR symbols you have been attuned to so as to maximize their healing potential.

You may invoke the string of beads at the beginning of a healing session in several ways, such as:

1. placing a string of beads in the palms of your hands,

Power Sandwich

2. placing a string of beads in each of the person's chakras, and/or

3. sending the string of beads through the crown chakra into the individual's heart center.

In each of these cases, your intention is that the energies be available throughout the session to be invoked according to your guidance on an as-needed basis. You may also call up a string of beads at any time during a session.

In the case of both a power sandwich and a string of beads, there is little chance of using too much power. This is because the recipient's higher self will draw only what is needed for the highest good of the person. Though you are amplifying many times the SSR energy available during the treatment, the recipient is not necessarily pulling in the maximum amount.

RELEASE OF PATTERNING

There is a specific application of Sei He Ki for the release and reprogramming of physical, mental and emotional patterns within the energy system and the cellular memory. In 1983, my first Reiki Master, John Harvey Gray, used the following technique to help me stop a three-pack-a-day smoking habit.

Each day for thirty days before I stopped smoking, John sent me from a distance (see Distance Healing section on the opposite page) various affirmations we had written together, including my stop date and the method I was going to use to quit smoking. We also checked in by telephone occasionally so that we could fine-tune the procedure as needed. Once my stop date arrived, we modified the affirmations accordingly, and he continued to send healing energy for another thirty days.

I have not smoked since October 1, 1983. Before John sent the energy to me, I had tried countless times to give up cigarettes with little success. Once I quit, I continued to go through a deep physical, emotional, mental and spiritual cleansing and clearing process for several years, which reflected letting go of the old patterning that had held the addiction in place.

Allow guidance to lead you in working with this process. Before beginning, be sure you understand what the client wishes to heal and how he or she desires to approach the healing. Devise one or more short, positive affirmations that are meaningful to the person to accomplish this purpose. The affirmations must be acceptable to the conscious mind as well as worded positively for the subconscious mind. A prayer may also be used along with sacred sound.

1. Invoke Cho Ku Rei "A" over the client's head and mentally repeat its name three times to bring in full power.

2. Place your left hand under the recipient's head with the fingertips at the base of the skull. Then sign Sei He Ki over the crown chakra or the third eye and mentally say Sei He Ki three times. Have the affirmations and prayers you will be using memorized or written on paper that is placed where you can easily read them.

3. Place your right hand across the crown or the forehead of the person, with the tips of your fingers pointed toward his or her left ear and the base of your palm toward the right ear. The moment both hands are in place, you are in direct contact with the left brain, the right brain and the cerebellum, which are directly linked to the conscious, subconscious and superconscious minds, respectively. This is an important responsibility. Whatever you think or say goes directly into these levels, so it is wise to be as clear and intentional as possible during this time.

4. With your hands in position as described above, call the individual's name in your mind three times, then repeat the affirmations and prayers three times either silently or aloud. My preference is aloud as this allows the client to hear the words which further reinforces the healing. If the client is willing, ask him or her to repeat the words aloud with you. Then hold the position for whatever length of time intuitively feels appropriate. Say "amen" or some other word or phrase to indicate

completion and to seal the opening to the conscious, subconscious and superconscious minds.

5. At the end of the session, give the person a copy of the affirmations and prayers and suggest that he or she repeat them several times a day to help reinforce and activate the healing process.

Using this same procedure, you may be guided to invoke Sei He Ki spontaneously during a session to infuse affirmations, sacred chants, tones and prayers into a person's entire energy system. This will likewise encourage the release of undesirable patterning and reprogram the cellular memory with higher light frequencies.

DISTANCE HEALING

Hon Sha Ze Sho Nen is used for sending a healing session over a distance. Be sure that you have the permission of the recipient before sending a distance healing. If you have been consciously asked by the person to send a healing, this is sufficient. Otherwise, you may ask permission of the person's higher self if you feel confident in your ability to accurately hear its reply.

If you receive a green light, then proceed with sending the distance healing. If you do not, universal law requires that you respect the person's wishes and not send the energy. This is important and should not be taken lightly because interfering with a person's free will can create undesirable consequences for you from a karmic standpoint.

If possible, ask the recipient to lie down and quietly meditate while you are sending a distance healing. This will empower the person to more fully participate in the healing process and may enhance his or her awareness of what is taking place during the session. The person will also be able to provide you with feedback about what took place. However, the effectiveness of distance healing is not affected by what the recipient is doing while you are sending the healing nor by his or her awareness of the process. Thus, the recipient can be engaged in any activity including work, sports or sleep.

The following procedure is suggested for sending a distance healing:

1. Create a quiet space where you can work uninterrupted by distractions such as television or a ringing telephone. Become quiet and meditative. You may also wish to play soft music in the background and have your physical space set up in the same manner as when you do in-person sessions.

2. Say the name of the person three times and visualize his or her energy in front of you. Place your hands over the recipient's forehead and third eye area and sign Hon Sha Ze Sho Nen once, saying its name three times. See the symbol melt into the forehead.

3. Place the person's energy in whatever space you are using for the session. For example, you can use the area where you usually give in-person sessions, such as on a massage table. You can also place a pillow on your lap and visualize the person in miniature on the pillow. Another option is visualizing each full-size body part on the pillow one at a time as you work on it. You can also make the recipient small enough to place him or her in the palms of your hands or use a doll, stuffed animal or photograph as a proxy.

4. Proceed with the energy work as usual, using the entire SSR matrix, angelic light weaving, toning and any of the SSR symbols you may intuitively be directed to apply.

5. When the session is complete, say "amen" or some other word or phrase to indicate completion and to close down the energetic connection to the recipient.

Once you are adept at distance healing, you may want to add more than one person at a time. However, be aware of any sense of dilution of power as you do this. Do not add people if you feel that the power level is adversely affected.

Energetic Strings and Cords

Sometimes during the course of a session you will come across areas within the physical and subtle bodies that are undesirably linked by energetic strings. For example, an old or lingering karmic thought form may still be connected to more than one area of the energy system, such as within the mental and emotional fields. Or you may be able to energetically unblock the liver by releasing fear held in the solar plexus that is connected through an energetic string to an old soul lesson also involving the liver. Perhaps there is a cool second chakra attached to a cool and closed heart chakra.

A powerful example of this healing technique is releasing a negative energetic connection between the heart and the sexual organs where a traumatic sexual event simultaneously closed down both areas. In this situation, the negative trauma in the lower chakras might need to be addressed prior to working on the heart chakra so that it will more easily release the connection to the lower fear vibrations. The energetic string between the areas can then be safely detached and the vitality of both regained. Finally, you can create a positive connection between the affected areas, developing an affirmation about loving relationships, for example, which you may send into the person's energy field as you close that area of work.

Energetic cords extending through our auric fields connect us to all forms of relationships. Barbara Brennan discusses five kinds of energetic cords in detail in her book *Light Emerging*. The first type—the soul cord—connects a person to his or her "original god connection" and monad. The second type connects a person's chakras to experiences from past lives. A third type is genetic, connecting the individual to his or her biological parents. The other two types of cords are relational and connect the person to his or her parents (not necessarily biological) and to other people.

Your attention to these energetic cords in order to untangle them, repair damage, change the flow from negative to positive energy or disconnect them completely often effects profound healing and welcome changes in the relationship being addressed, be it with the Source of ALL LOVE, the client's past lives, or another person.

I have found that disconnecting cords completely can be advisable when a relationship is over or after a death if the person seeking healing has been unable to move forward with his or her life for a prolonged amount of time after the loss. The technique can also be highly beneficial when there are channels open in your client's fields that permit negative psychic energy and debris from another person to continue affecting and intruding on the client in an unwelcome way. The goal is to allow the individual to fully and energetically move away from the other person and reestablish his or her own energetic boundaries, integrity and wholeness.

If you are guided to suggest removing one or more cords, obtain permission from your client and proceed with compassion and understanding, since emotions such as sadness, grief or even anger may be triggered. Ask for your client's full cooperation and participation in the activity. He or she must truly want and be ready to let go of the other person. You must also intuitively obtain permission from the higher self of the individual on the other end of the cord.

After you introduce the option of removing a cord, your client may need additional time to consider and proceed with the removal process. Any doubt or reluctance on the client's part is an indication that it may be too soon. Respect those times when an individual is not ready to clear an area of the physical or subtle bodies while you continue providing gentle encouragement and support. It is a waste of effort to detach the cords when full readiness and intention are not present on the client's part as the cords will most likely reattach themselves.

Part of the process of coming to readiness might include encouraging the client to speak aloud whatever he or she needs to say to the other person as a means of bringing closure to the relationship. If words are difficult, toning or making other sounds often helps to shift the energy. See the section on Sound Healing, below.

When you pull a cord out, take care to remove it entirely using your intuition to guide you. Portions of it may have reached beyond the chakra or area where it entered similar to the energetic strings discussed above that trail through several subtle bodies. If you have the permission of the absent person's higher self, remove the other end of the cord thoroughly as well. Saturate the entire cord with clear light and ask Archangel Michael to carry it away for disposal. If the absent person's higher self has refused permission for removal, take the cord out of your client, saturate the exposed end with clear light and lovingly send it back to the other person. Fill the spaces emptied by the cord with clear light.

Sometimes it is necessary to cut an active cord that is resisting being pulled out. When this is the case, employ the use of a large pair of scissors by visualizing them slicing the cord all the way through. It then will likely be a simple procedure to clean the end of the cord out of the etheric body. Another method of removing a resistant cord is to completely dissolve it using clear light.

Sealing Auric Leaks

If you come across a cool space or hole within the person's energy field, you may have found what is called an auric leak. These leaks are weak spots within the auric field created by physical, emotional, mental or spiritual traumas and events from past and present lifetimes. Auric leaks allow vital life force energy to drain out, depleting the entire energy system. Auric damage can be caused by taking illegal drugs as well as certain prescription formulas such as sleeping pills, diet pills, pain killers and muscle relaxers. Smoking and other substance abuse also causes leaks.

This kind of imbalance needs to be repaired, sealed and smoothed out. There are several methods for this, including simply focusing your mind and third eye upon the area to reestablish its natural vibrational pattern.

You may also scan your hand gently across the area and use angelic light weaving to assist you. Make sure the area is completely infused with light energy and rewoven before moving on. You may wish to return to that location later in the session to make sure the area has remained sealed.

Sound Healing

I was introduced to the power of healing with sound in the early 1980s when I attended a group that chanted sacred mantras. I loved the chanting and was so taken by its positive effects that I played tapes in my car on long drives, chanting the entire time. I found the melodies and the repetitive nature of the chants to be soothing and nurturing. Chanting sacred sounds was also very comforting and infused my being with spiritual frequencies that helped me feel closer to the Divine and activated the release of much sadness, anger and other emotions. I continue doing the chanting to this day.

A key element of Patrick Zeigler's approach to healing with SKHM is the use of sound. This includes a great deal of toning and overtoning. Toning is the use of the human voice to produce sounds that are cleansing, harmonizing and healing. Overtoning is toning a basic note which can then produce accompanying lower and higher sounds known as harmonics or overtones. These are sounds that are in a mathematical ratio with the basic note.

Becoming highly skilled at overtoning can require much practice. Yet when a person begins to simply tone and allows him or herself to flow with the sound wanting to emerge, harmonics are often produced spontaneously without formal instruction in overtoning. This also occurs when people tone together as a group.

Toning was a prominent part of my first weekend experience with Patrick in 1997. I was impressed with its healing effects on everyone, especially the way toning dealt with energy blocks and constrictions with relative ease. I also could not help but notice how toning could be used to saturate a person's entire being with the SSR and SKHM healing frequencies, as well as the healing vibration of particular spiritual qualities such as forgiveness, love, joy and compassion. I immediately began incorporating toning into my healing work with clients and myself. I also read several books and attended workshops on sound healing.

When using sound during a healing session, I ask for higher guidance and invite whatever sound or sounds are needed by the person to emerge through my voice. Sometimes the tones seem dissonant and unpleasant sounding; at other times they are quite exquisite and pleasing to the ear. I have found that the unpleasant tones are most useful when opening and shifting an energy block out of the energy system, while the pleasing sounds complete the release process and bring forth the spiritual healing quality or qualities most needed by the recipient at that moment. Sometimes the sounds may also be expressed in the form of syllables and words suggestive of a Native American tongue or an ancient or foreign language.

Often I invite the client to tone along with me, making the effects of the toning even more powerful than when I tone by myself. I encourage the person to move his or her consciousness into the area being addressed and give voice to the sound or sounds that reflect what needs to be expressed. The client's sounds may be similar to or different from those I am toning and may also include words or syllables.

At times I find myself bringing my mouth close to a particular area on the recipient's body or placing my hand on that spot and conducting the sound through my hand. At other times, I tone further away from the body. I also find that sometimes my throat becomes constricted during the process of toning, which mirrors the energetics of what is being released by the recipient. As my throat opens up again and the sound becomes clearer, this indicates the area is now unblocked and opening up. To further cleanse and purify the area, I follow up with toning whatever sounds I am guided to use to infuse the area with higher sound frequencies and qualities.

I also use sound when I teach workshops or give talks. Once again, I simply open my voice to bring forward whatever tones would be beneficial for both the group as a whole and for individuals within the group. This invokes the flow of the SSR and SKHM healing energy in the group setting. It is also an effective and powerful way to foster group cohesion and harmony and clear any energetics that may be distracting or incongruent with the purpose of the gathering. I often invite members of the audience to join in the toning, as this moves the process to a deeper level.

You do not have to have a beautiful singing voice or formal voice training in order to be highly effective in using toning. I have merely allowed my voice to be used as a channel for bringing through those tones and sounds that would be beneficial. Give yourself permission to let go of all fears, insecurities and self-consciousness about how others might react to the sounds you make. Tune into the highest levels of consciousness and ask for the healing energy to flow through your voice. A wonderful secondary benefit of toning for others is that you will also be clearing and healing yourself.

The wise choice of music for use during a healing session can also greatly assist in the process. I ask for divine guidance when choosing what to play. Sometimes the music is soothing and calming. At other times, it is more lively and rhythmic. Occasionally, I am directed not to play any music. In addition, I have incorporated the use of the crystal singing bowls, tuning forks and Tibetan bells into my practice.

Chanting sounds in the form of a mantra can also be highly beneficial. Mantras are sacred sounds that can stimulate deep healing and evoke focused awareness of altered states of consciousness when repeated many times. For example, you might chant the mantra ALL LOVE to open up the flow of the SKHM energy stream within yourself. You may also suggest that a client chant the mantra during a session and/or as part of an ongoing meditation practice.

Another divine mantra often associated with the SKHM energy stream is "Sa Sekhem Sahu." In his book *The Goddess Sekhmet,* Robert Masters explains the meaning of this mantra. "Sa" is the breath of life, the energizing force by which everything is given life. "Sekhem" means power or might. This power allows the individual to operate in the human dimensions as well as in the higher dimensions. "Sahu" is symbolic of the attainment of the highest subtle body, which is the realized human. In short, Masters translates the meaning of this mantra as follows:

Sa	*The Breath of Life*
Sekhem	*The Sacred Might*
Sahu	*The Realized Human*

Please refer to *The Goddess Sekhmet* for additional information regarding this sacred mantra, including how it can be used during meditation.

Sound healing is based on several principles, including resonance, rhythm, melody, harmony, pitch and timbre. It is not within the scope of this Guidebook to include a full technical discussion of these principles, but if you wish to delve more deeply into this growing field, please refer to the Bibliography.

Using Conscious Breathwork or Rebirthing

I often use conscious breathwork (also known as rebirthing) together with SSR during a session. The energy of the breath is one of the most natural and inborn resources available for awakening one's innate healing ability and infusing divine light frequencies and vital energy into the human energy system.

Conscious breathwork is a loving and gentle, yet powerful holistic approach to healing that works well with SSR for releasing and clearing suppressed physical, mental, emotional and spiritual blocks and negative patterning that result from a person's life experiences, including past lives. The rhythm of conscious breathing is gentle, with the inhalation connected to the exhalation in a continuous cycle and with total relaxation on the exhalation.

For optimum health and well-being, a person's breath must flow smoothly throughout all of the energy pathways, enlivening the body. Shallow and restricted breathing is very common and is an effective way for the body to suppress the experience of traumas, anger, stress, fear, anxiety, sadness or other physical or emotional pain. This reaction is part of the body's natural defense system and can be helpful during times of crisis. But any longstanding, uncorrected imbalances in the flow of the breath or life force will usually result in blocks that create physical, mental and emotional fatigue and illness and eventually, perhaps even death.

To experience conscious breathwork, find a qualified rebirther and consider completing a series of sessions for your personal healing. The rebirther can also help you find resources for learning how to become a rebirther should this be a technique you want to include in your healing toolkit. The Bibliography contains several references for books on the subject.

Closing Spiral

About ten to fifteen minutes before the session ends, I usually ask the person if there is anything else he or she feels is incomplete or needs to be dealt with before closing. Sometimes I word it by requesting that the client do a scan of his or her body and energy field to see if there is any area that needs a bit more attention. This provides the client with practice in self-awareness and speaking those needs aloud. I also find that opening this opportunity and using the remaining time to deal with those needs allows the recipient to feel a sense of completion even though he or she may not have come to final resolution of the issue being addressed.

To complete the session, use a closing spiral, moving your hand in the opposite or counterclockwise spin from when you opened the session (soul star, Earth star, crown chakra, root chakra, third eye chakra, sacral chakra, throat chakra, solar plexus chakra, heart chakra). As you complete the spiral and return to the heart chakra, take the receiver's hands and stack them over his or her heart in an intertwining pattern with your hands (first one of your client's hands, then yours on top, then your client's other hand, and finally your other hand). Hold this position for the amount of time that feels appropriate.

Then light weave a spiraling infinity or figure eight pattern from the top of the client's head to beneath the feet and back to the top of the head, with the center or crossover point at the heart. I also light weave the ankh into the energy field. After completing these patterns, you may sweep the entire energy field from top to bottom several times, starting above the head and moving to below the feet, shaking off or gently brushing the left and right hands together with the intention of closing all of the energy bodies while invoking a protective grid of light. Place your hands about three or four inches above the body for this sweeping process.

End the session with prayers of gratitude. Suggest the person remain lying down with his or her eyes closed for a short time until an inner prompting is received indicating it is time to return to regular waking consciousness. Usually a person will come back in just a few minutes.

Session Follow-up

Make sure the recipient's energy field is smooth and sealed and that the person is well grounded before leaving. Once in a while, this may require a glass of water and perhaps a snack. Be sure that both the recipient and you drink plenty of water in the hours immediately following a session to flush out of the system the toxins that have been dislodged during the healing. You may also wish to suggest a cleansing bath as discussed in the section called Preparing Yourself, on page 62.

It is important to make your client aware of the possible aftereffects of an energy healing so he or she better understands how to deal with them. This is necessary because the SSR energy stream often initiates a process whereby built up energetic debris and toxins are flushed from one or more of the physical, emotional, mental and spiritual levels. There is also a simultaneous integration, alignment and balancing taking place at every level of the person's being. Please see the section entitled The Heart of Healing, beginning on page 35 for a more detailed discussion of the healing process. Also see the section entitled Professional Standards of Care, on page 86.

Be sure to let your client know of your availability for follow-up conversation and in-person or distance healing in order to provide additional support for whatever he or she may be experiencing.

How you approach and understand the healing process will influence how often you recommend that a client comes to see you. I have found that most of the time, it is not necessary for a client to come weekly unless he or she wants to do some very concentrated and focused healing work or is in the middle of a crisis period. I usually find that the client knows when it is time for another session. I also ask for inner guidance on the matter of timing and encourage the client to do the same. In some circumstances, I am guided to suggest a series of sessions spaced apart by two or three weeks. This allows integration time between sessions and is also kind to the client's pocketbook.

Working with Animals

Many animals love SSR and can greatly benefit from both energy healing and the attunements. This includes dogs, cats, horses and other pets. Approach an animal with compassion to establish trust and rapport and to allow the animal to sense your intention to assist. Some will allow you to directly touch them while others will not. In the latter case, you may beam the healing energy from your hands to the animal from a few inches away from the body. You may even send a distance healing using the same procedure used for humans.

I have also used SSR to assist animals in passing on. These situations usually have arisen when I have found an injured animal while outside walking in the woods or in my yard, and it is clear the animal is in the death process. In these cases, I have beamed the energy to the animal from a few inches away, soothingly blessed its spirit and intuitively guided it on its way.

My cat Ganesha has injured himself many times. Once he was bitten by a snake. Another time he fell across something sharp which created an abscess in his tummy area. Both injuries required surgery. I was able to use SSR both before and after surgery to help him heal more quickly.

Even when healthy, Ganesha loves to soak up the SSR energy. On many occasions he has been known to forego a precious day outside to attend an SSR class, where he proudly takes a seat just like the students and sits with us for hours. While present in these classes, I attuned him to all seven facets of SSR. Ganesha also loves to give SSR and regularly assists during healing sessions by showing up and interacting with clients in various ways, including lying on top of them and placing his paws in certain areas.

I have learned to intuitively follow and trust what Ganesha is doing, which has provided me with valuable clues as to how to proceed with a session. One time at the beginning of a session, he kept sniffing near and around the client's right hip area for an extended period of time. Within a few minutes of my treating the area, the client announced that she needed to excuse herself to use the bathroom. The heavy constipation she had been experiencing for several days seemed to be loosening up. Needless to say, I was most impressed.

In another example, I was at a point in a session where I was absolutely baffled and did not have any idea of where to go next. Ganesha then walked across the client's thighs. Something told me that this was my answer, so I began working in this area. Shortly thereafter, there was an almost audible release of old stored energy that had been trapped in the legs. The client described feeling a kind of a"whoosh," which was followed by a steady flow of unconditional love and peace into her body. The client later reported significant improvement in her situation, which not surprisingly had to do with moving forward and making a desired change in her life.

I know of many other practitioners and teachers who have had similar experiences with their animals. Be open to the assistance that is available to you at all levels, including from our animal friends and teachers, as they are often more tuned in to our vibrations than we give them credit for.

PART FOUR:
On Being a Healing Practitioner and Teacher

Qualities and Values of a Healing Practitioner and Teacher

There are many beneficial and desirable qualities, characteristics, values and practices that will help you feel good about yourself and assure your continuing growth and success as a healing practitioner and teacher of SSR and SKHM. These encompass your personal qualities and values, professional standards and skills, ethical considerations, legal issues and how you honor yourself as a healer as well as the healing process itself.

Because we are each a "work in process," it is not my intention to imply a need to be perfect. Rather, the purpose of this section is to help you be aware of the various factors that may influence your ability to work successfully with others as well as how you feel about yourself as a healing practitioner and teacher of SSR and SKHM.

The following list also provides guidelines for a prospective client or student when considering a potential healing practitioner or teacher. The SSR and SKHM energy stream itself will not be affected by how clear the practitioner or teacher is. In some cases, however, the unhealed aspects of the individual's own energy system and life can create undesirable and unbalanced interactions in the practitioner/client or teacher/student relationship. Just because SSR and SKHM are forms of spiritual healing does not mean that ego dynamics such as denial, competitiveness and being judgmental cannot become involved. Use discernment at all times in making your choice.

I strongly suggest that practitioners and teachers use this list as a starting point for an ongoing process of self-evaluation that includes goal-setting, personal healing and taking action to make changes in those areas that need enhancement and improvement. A healing practitioner and teacher of SSR and SKHM:

- Is actively committed to his or her personal healing process, which includes healing the shadow self and taking personal responsibility for all that takes place in his or her life.
- Feels an inner calling to be of service.
- Creates a safe and open atmosphere for clients where all possibilities exist.
- Respects the confidentiality of all information obtained during sessions and classes.
- Trusts in the abundance and ALL LOVE of the universe.
- Recognizes his or her own basic goodness and strength as well as that of the client.

- Empowers the recipient to tap into and awaken his or her own healing resources.
- Honors the recipient by asking permission to send healing energy.
- Has no expectation of a particular outcome, asking for the highest good of all concerned.
- Develops an inner alignment of the lower will with the Higher Will by cultivating an attitude of "Thy Will be Done" and "I Will to Will Thy Will."
- Recognizes that it is not possible to heal or "save" another person as an individual must take responsibility for his or her own healing.
- Has an open and compassionate heart.
- Develops non-judgmental listening and communication skills.
- Consistently asks for, listens to, accepts and acts on inner guidance.
- Sets aside his or her ego and personality needs and is fully present in the moment.
- Supports and empowers others in finding their own answers.
- Teaches by example.
- Encourages and teaches clients and students to directly connect to their own power and the Source of ALL LOVE.
- Is knowledgeable about SSR and SKHM and actively works with the energy stream on a regular basis to gain experience and understanding.
- Is knowledgeable about the human energy system.
- Is knowledgeable about the healing process and techniques that support it.
- Is knowledgeable about learning styles and effective teaching methods.
- Has an ever-expanding capacity and thirst for new knowledge.
- Regularly attends classes and seminars that enhance professional qualifications, training, experience and skills.
- Treats clients, students, professional colleagues and him or herself with the greatest respect.
- Encourages harmony and friendly cooperation among all practitioners and teachers regardless of lineage or affiliation.
- Sets aside time for him or herself for adequate rest and relaxation by planning days off, vacations, meditative time and play time.
- Is open and honest in advertising and stating education, qualifications, level of training and background.
- Informs clients and students that though SSR and SKHM complement many modalities of treatment, they do not guarantee a "cure" and are not substitute for appropriate medical and psychological care and treatment.
- Refrains from diagnosing or prescribing unless licensed to do so by the state or jurisdiction in which he or she practices or teaches.
- Knows the limits of those conditions and issues he or she is qualified to address with clients.
- Makes referrals to qualified health care professionals when needed.
- Is familiar and complies with the requirements of any and all laws and regulations of the state or jurisdiction where he or she is located, including professional and business licensing, insurance regulations and tax implications.
- Obtains permission to use the copyrighted and non-copyrighted information and materials of others and gives appropriate credit to the originator.

I believe the single most essential quality of a practitioner and teacher of SSR and SKHM is actively committing to his or her own healing process, which includes healing the shadow self and taking personal responsibility for all that takes place in his or her life. Understanding that the outer world is a reflection of your inner state helps in appreciating that the people and situations in your life offer many opportunities for deep healing of core issues.

Be willing to look inside yourself whenever you notice any form of "negativity" cropping up in your thoughts and life. Consider that it may be a positive signal for you to learn to accept, forgive and release to the light those unhealed shadow parts of yourself that have been kept hidden. Create a network of support people to call on when you require assistance, including seeking professional help when your need is great.

Clients and students will mirror and reflect back your own shadow patterns, which must be cleared. A practitioner and teacher cannot be fully present and available if his or her own issues are getting in the way. In addition, doing your personal healing work provides much useful knowledge about the healing process that can be of great value when working with others. Sharing your personal healing experiences and the related lessons with clients and students when appropriate also enriches and enhances the experience for all concerned.

Each of us is a beautiful tapestry and a "work in process." Take care not to fall into the ego trap where you feel you have "arrived" and no longer need to do your own healing work. I have observed many who attempt to make what I call a "spiritual bypass." They focus primarily on the higher aspects of themselves while ignoring all the other levels of their existence.

Part of the process of healing the shadow self also includes directly examining your motivations for wanting to be of service. They may not all be altruistic and benevolent when held up to closer scrutiny. For example, a person may be inspired to be of service by being an addictions counselor, yet behind this is a need for validation of the counselor's worthiness. Other underlying factors might include the need for control, power, fame or love. An excellent book that will help you in exploring such motivations as well as understanding the various dimensions of service work is *Born to Serve* by Susan Trout.

A common issue found in the shadow self for practitioners and teachers is their feelings of unworthiness

to carry the divine light of the SSR and SKHM energy stream. A practitioner or teacher may also be concerned that his or her degree of learning and training is not enough when compared with others. Both of these experiences are another way of saying, "I am not worthy" and "I am not enough." If feelings of unworthiness are strong, consider addressing and focusing on them as part of your ongoing personal healing process.

An example from my life regarding healing a shadow issue grew out of the birthing process I have gone through in writing this Guidebook. What I first perceived as a simple and quick writing exercise turned into a major project that lasted close to three years in part due to my unwillingness to envision myself as an author with something worthwhile to say about any subject matter, including SSR and SKHM.

I also encountered issues about aligning myself with the divine plan for this Guidebook along the way. I found I had to let go of my need to control the outcome and learn to trust that there was a right and perfect timing for its completion. More than once I set a finish date, made promises to my students and was then unable to keep my word. This upset me tremendously as I am rarely unreliable in this regard.

As I delved inside myself for the answer to my difficulties, I discovered yet another reason why I was dragging my feet: a strong reluctance to face a core fear of being worthy to claim my full God/Goddess-given power, step out more visibly into the public domain and get on with the next stage of the universal light work I am here to be a part of.

While I was writing early in the morning of New Year's Eve 1998, I hit an all-too-familiar wall for what seemed like the umpteenth time. I prayed for inspiration. Later on that day, I came across and reread as though for the first time a portion of Nelson Mandela's inaugural speech quoted by him from *A Return to Love* by Marianne Williamson. The words brought tears to my eyes and struck a deep chord inside of me, heartening my soul and giving me the courage and strength

I needed to heal my issues and move forward. I share these often-quoted words in the hope they will be meaningful to you as well:

Our deepest fear is not that we are inadequate.
Our deepest fear is that we are powerful beyond measure.
It is our light, not our darkness, that most frightens us.
We ask ourselves, Who am I to be brilliant, gorgeous, talented, fabulous?
Actually, who are you not to be?
You are a child of God.
Your playing small doesn't serve the world.
There's nothing enlightened about shrinking so that other people won't feel insecure around you.
We are all meant to shine, as children do.
We were born to make manifest the glory of God that is within us.
It's not just in some of us; it's in everyone.
And as we let our own light shine, we unconsciously give other people permission to do the same.
As we're liberated from our own fear,
Our presence automatically liberates others.

Instantly, my concerns began to melt away. Being in alignment with the Higher Will was much easier and time became less of an issue. I turned the Guidebook and my authorship of it over to the Source of ALL LOVE and, not surprisingly, the Guidebook began to write itself. As well, I felt a much stronger connection to the Source and felt more at peace with my role as a vehicle for this Guidebook to come into form.

This example from my life emphasizes the fact that one of the greatest soul-expanding lessons you can learn from being a channel of the SSR and SKHM energy stream is to embody within yourself the knowledge and experience that this form of service work is an extension of your direct connection with the Source of ALL LOVE and is very likely a part of your soul purpose. Personal healing of this core shadow issue will enhance your ability to be a clear conduit for assisting others to likewise remember their divine truth and connection with the Source of ALL LOVE.

Though the healing process can at times be difficult and painful, the rewards are enormous. As healing progresses, the practitioner and teacher is freed up to gradually become a clearer channel for the living light energy of SSR and SKHM. Living in alignment with your highest truth and the qualities and values listed and discussed above becomes easier and easier and is a natural extension of your ever-deepening personal healing work. The truth of who a person is provides a powerful model to those who come for healing sessions and classes and encourages them to do the same through the example set by the practitioner and teacher. See the section entitled The Heart of Healing, on page 35 for more information on the healing process.

Attend well to your physical, emotional, mental and spiritual levels so that all components of your inner and outer life reflect this balance, integration and grounding. The result will be greater and greater levels of consistency in your thoughts, emotions, words and actions, enabling you to truly "walk your talk" honestly and in full integrity.

Establishing a Healing Practice

Decisions, Decisions, Decisions

I have found the most important question to answer when deciding whether to open a healing practice is, "Who am I?" Your answer will help define what you want to create and guide you in making the many choices that will present themselves. If your answer has anything to do with healing, you may be heading in the direction of opening some form of healing practice.

Many who receive SSR attunements or work with SKHM, however, do not feel a calling in the early stages to actively promote themselves as healers. Rather, as they begin to feel ready, they informally get the word out to their family and friends and practice on them to gain experience working with the energy.

Practitioners may also gain more experience by participating in occasional or regular healing work in volunteer settings, such as hospitals, churches or various service and spiritual organizations. Some teachers sponsor regular healing groups and circles where practitioners can offer their services to those who come to receive healing.

In answering the question "Who am I?" it is important to note that healing does not always have to be hands-on, as in a typical energy session. A person may well know that he or she is a healer, yet finds another way of expressing this gift such as through painting or singing. In such cases, the healing energy touches the hearts and souls of those who are open as they gaze upon the artwork or listen to the song. Others may express their healing gifts in the preparation of wholesome foods or in their gardening work.

In many ways, it makes no difference whether you ever formally open a healing practice. Once you have deeply tapped into the universal flow of the SSR and SKHM energy stream, it is a part of you, and you are forever changed. You become an instrument of healing for those you come in contact with, even in the most casual way no matter the activity, be it work or play.

If you are headed in the direction of being an active healing practitioner and possibly opening a practice, you must decide on many essential details—what kinds of services to provide, your style and approach to healing, what kinds of clients you want to work with, the length of sessions, how much to charge for each service and where to see clients.

You will want to furnish your healing room with an adjustable massage table and other accessories such as plants, books, artwork, furniture, stereo or CD player and whatever else helps to create a healing environment that is safe, peaceful, calming and supportive of both the client's and your needs.

Another decision involves whether to work full or part-time. For many new practitioners, there is often a transition period where they find it financially necessary to continue earning an income in more traditional work settings while establishing and building their healing practices.

Professional Standards of Care

Professional standards of care are codes of conduct that a person is required to follow when offering services to clients, consumers or customers. Such standards exist for many traditional professions such as medical doctors, nurses, psychotherapists, members of the clergy, attorneys and public accountants. These standards vary from profession to profession and are decided by legislative and regulatory authorities, professional organizations and experts, as well as through exercising common sense.

Standards of care have also been established for certain complementary and alternative healing professions such as naturopathic doctors, chiropractors, acupuncturists and massage therapists. However, the creation of such guidelines for more recently emerging healing professions such as body workers and energy healers as of the time of this writing has not been as clear cut depending on the state in which you are practicing and whether a recognized professional organization exists for the profession in question.

The following general discussion of the issue is offered by Karen L. Meengs, Esq. in *The Goddess As Entrepreneur: Right-Brained Tools for Left-Brained Businesses©,* a course given in four segments on various legal, financial and practical aspects of being a solo practitioner and business owner. In the handouts provided in this seminar series and in the tapes of the series, Ms. Meengs discusses certain professional standards of care and legal duties owed to a client. These include:

- To use standards of care acceptable to the profession of which you are a member.

- To refer a person to others when his or her problem is beyond your capabilities, skills, training and expertise.

- To refrain from making misrepresentations or claims that go beyond your capabilities, skills, training and expertise.

- To furnish adequate information to a client that allows him or her to make an informed decision about whether to receive a specific form of care.

- To document pertinent information about the client.

With regard to these general guidelines, it is highly recommended that you consult the laws and regulations of the particular state in which you are setting up a healing practice to be sure you are in compliance with any existing standards of care for your profession. In addition, you may wish to become a member of any applicable professional organizations and implement their standards of care. If you are not licensed, you also want to be sure not to overstep your boundaries in terms of the state's legal definitions of what is considered the practice of medicine and/or psychotherapy, including any laws that define which professions are allowed to physically touch the body.

The next guideline discussed by Ms. Meengs relates to providing information to a person that allows him or her to make an informed decision about whether to receive a specific form of care such as an SSR healing session. In this connection, Appendix VIII contains a Sample SSR Client Consent Form that includes information about SSR and a disclaimer about the kind of services you are providing when doing an SSR session. The sample form also acquaints the person with your administrative policies relating to length of sessions, your fee structure, contingencies such as cancelled, missed or forgotten appointments, arriving late for appointments and bank charges for returned checks.

The consent form would typically be given to a person at his or her first visit and then signed in duplicate before you would proceed with the session. One copy is for the client and the other is for your files. **Please revise this form to reflect your particular state's laws as well as your individual circumstances.**

Ms. Meengs goes on to say that a client's file should include such information as the person's name, address, work and home telephone numbers, e-mail address, fax number and date of birth. The file should document information as to why the person has come to see you, including background information about the problem and any previous experience with any form of energy work. Make regular entries into a dated log of brief notes that cover what took place during a session, the services you have furnished and the client's response. Be sure that these notes include any recommendations you have made to the person and follow-up notations as to whether these recommendations have been implemented by him or her. As well, note cancelled or missed appointments in the file. You will also want to review the file immediately prior to your next session to help establish continuity and flow in your ongoing healing work with the person.

It is also strongly recommended that you keep your client records confidential even if there is no law on record-keeping applicable to your area of practice.

Disclosure to anyone of client information is inappropriate and is a violation of the client's trust in you. Besides being considered unethical in many professions, such disclosure erodes both the safety of your sessions and your professional integrity. Note, however, that some professionals such as psychotherapists actually have a duty to disclose under certain circumstances such as suspected child abuse or where the life of the client or another person is in danger. **Once again, check your state laws relative to confidentiality requirements as they often vary from state to state and from profession to profession.**

A Sample SSR Client Summary Form based on the preceding is included in Appendix IX. Fill out this form for each and every session with a client to create a running log of your sessions. Also use this form to record relevant information from any telephone conversations you have with the client between sessions or for distance healings that you perform on behalf of the client. Use additional sheets of paper if necessary. **Please note that this form should be revised to reflect the laws of your state and your individual circumstances.**

Marketing Your Services

From a business standpoint, you must also decide how to market your services. This is sometimes the most difficult part of having a practice because many practitioners have not learned how to express who they are in words, both aloud and on paper. I have found that having a business card and a brochure describing the services I offer has been very important for two key reasons. One is that deciding what to include in them has helped me define who I am in this regard. The second is that people seeking healing services and attunements usually like to have something tangible to read and absorb to help them choose the practitioner and teacher who is right for them.

Keeping your brochure and card up-to-date to reflect your evolving work is also essential so that others are aware of your current offerings. I have had at least five or six different versions of my brochure and business card in the last three years. The people who follow your work will want to hear about how you are expanding and growing.

Regularly advertising in newspapers and magazines read by potential clients is also valuable. Even though initially it is sometimes hard to gauge whether such advertising is successful, having your name out there on a regular basis eventually pays off. I have been amazed at the number of people I have met for the first time who, upon learning my name, have exclaimed, "Oh, you are Diane Shewmaker! I've seen your advertising and have been meaning to call you." I have had the most success with publications geared toward those who are holistically, spiritually and metaphysically oriented.

You may also advertise your services by creating a website on the Internet, taking care to register it with the most widely used search engines. You will be surprised to find the places from which people contact you—from all over the world to as close as your own back yard. I have made many wonderful contacts through the Internet that have resulted in new business as well as in making new friends.

I have participated in many holistic and metaphysical health fairs and expos over the years by having a booth where I provided sample sessions and gave out literature to attendees. Many fairs and expos also offer opportunities to give free workshops. I have always taken advantage of these since they have helped me develop teaching skills, and because personal contact is often the key to attracting clients and students. Cultivating personal relationships is also important in developing referrals from others who feel good about recommending your services to their family members, friends and coworkers.

Attending health fairs and expos to see firsthand how others are setting up their booths and presenting themselves in their literature and advertising is also useful. This can help with inspiring you to find your own perfect form of expressing the services you have to offer. Relevant magazines and newspapers are also a rich source of information. Be careful, however, not to copy others' materials, not only because of possible copyright violations but also because it is not being respectful of their creation. There are countless ways to communicate who you are without the need to imitate others. You have the inner resources within your own creative wellspring.

I maintain a mailing list on my computer and do two to three mailings a year including such items as my brochure and business card, flyers for scheduled workshops, a calendar of public appearances and travel plans, plus a cover letter informing the reader of any new services that have been added. I have built my list from contacts made by people responding to my advertising or who I meet at expos and other events, including classes that I teach.

Other possible places to advertise, and provide your healing services are the offices of holistic doctors and other health care providers such as acupuncturists and massage therapists, retirement facilities, metaphysical stores, health food stores and health spas. The people who own and frequent these places are also resources for finding out about newspapers, magazines and expos in your area.

Accounting Records

Good accounting records are a must for tax purposes and for providing you with valuable information about the financial standing of your practice. You will want to create ledgers that accurately reflect your income and expenses and update them regularly while keeping detailed files that contain the actual invoices and backup paperwork for the ledgers. Many computer programs available today are excellent for creating these ledgers.

The U. S. Internal Revenue Service and the taxing authority in your state have regulations about valid expenses and deductions that you must document in order to be in compliance. Even though I have a background in accounting, federal tax law and preparing tax returns, I have found it beneficial to hire a certified public accountant who can answer my tax questions throughout the year and prepare my tax returns.

Legal and Business Aspects

For more information on the legal and business aspects of a healing arts practice, contact Karen L. Meengs, Esq. about her course *The Goddess as Entrepreneur.* Her address, telephone and e-mail are: 746-10 Walker Road, Great Falls, Virginia 22066, 888-447-0024, EsquetteJD@aol.com.

Learning to Trust One Day at a Time

Taking care of the many aspects of creating and maintaining a healing practice can seem daunting, especially in the beginning. But there is no substitute for moving forward with your vision and plans one day at a time while gradually picking up the skills and confidence you need. No one, including your SSR and SKHM teacher, can give you this self-assurance, whether you study with him or her for one day, one year or ten years.

I did not create the success of my healing practice overnight. In fact, since I first learned Reiki in the early 1980's, I have gone through several difficult stages during which I have doubted myself and my capabilities, first as a practitioner, then as a teacher, and most recently as a writer. I would still be at square one, depressed and upset with myself, had I not been willing to take each step along the way as guided by my heart, while working through and healing each of my fears as they came up. I strongly recommend reading *Jonathan Livingston Seagull* by Richard Bach for inspiration in overcoming obstacles.

Though ultimately you must learn to walk this path directed from your inner core, you do not have to do it alone. You can find encouragement and ideas on how to proceed by talking with people who have walked the same path ahead of you. You can also reach out to others for support when in need. As well, your spirit guides and angels, the ascended masters and the Source of ALL LOVE are always with you. As you learn to connect more completely with them, they will provide a wealth of unlimited inspiration, support, empowerment and guidance.

You may also count on the SKHM and SSR energy stream to teach you about itself and how to draw upon its healing resources even beyond what is included in this Guidebook. You will become a stronger and clearer channel the more you consciously work with the energy for healing others and yourself.

From the earliest days of consciously addressing my personal healing beginning over twenty years ago, I somehow knew from the deepest part of my soul that it was essential for me to walk this sacred path despite my countless misgivings, doubts, anxieties and financial concerns. The following passage by W.H. Murray as quoted in *To See Differently* by Susan Trout has been inspirational and helpful to me in staying on course:

Until one is committed
There is hesitancy, the chance to draw back,
Always ineffectiveness.
Concerning all acts of initiative (and creation),
There is one elementary truth,
The ignorance of which kills countless ideas
And splendid plans:
That the moment one definitely commits oneself,
then Providence moves too.
All sorts of things occur to help one
That would never otherwise have occurred.
A whole stream of events issues from the decision,
Raising in one's favour all manner
Of unforeseen incidents and meetings
And material assistance,
Which no man could have dreamt
Would have come his way.
I have learned a deep respect for one of Goethe's couplets:
"Whatever you can do, or dream you can, begin it.
Boldness has genius, power and magic in it."

Opening to all possibilities and allowing the stages of my healing journey to unfold one by one has required me to learn to listen to, trust and have faith in the inner voice of the Source of ALL LOVE and my guides and angels, who have all encouraged and loved me throughout the entire process. As each stage transitioned into the next, I have had to be willing to let go of that which had become comfortable and stretch my wings and fly into the unknown.

This Guidebook would truly have not seen the light of day had I been unwilling to say "yes" to my innermost heart's desires and learn to be in alignment with my soul purpose and reason for being. This is an ongoing process.

As this Guidebook is completed, I have followed inner guidance to move with my husband to Oregon from my birthplace in Washington, D.C. where I lived my entire life until now. I have some idea of what lies ahead, yet in many ways I do not. Part of me wants to play it safe, yet thankfully I have reached the place where most of me is ready and willing to soar beyond my wildest dreams. And so here I go once again—brushing off my wings, taking to the air and trusting, trusting, trusting.

Becoming a Teacher

When I was first attuned to Reiki, I had no idea where I was going with it. I only knew I was drawn to the energy both as a receiver and as a student, learning to apply it to help others through the healing process. It was not until 1995 when I became a Reiki Master and simultaneously received my first Seichim attunements that I understood for certain I was going to become a teacher of Reiki and Seichim. At the time, I already had been teaching workshops and training sessions in attitudinal healing, ascension, finding your soul purpose, rebirthing and other holistic and metaphysical topics.

I began teaching Reiki and Seichim shortly after receiving the Reiki Master and Seichim I-IV attunements. Initially, I co-taught introductory workshops with my teacher at various locations including health and metaphysical expos. I also taught classes on my own in all three degrees of Reiki and Facets I-III of Seichim. By 1996, I had completed the remaining Seichim attunements and began teaching all seven facets of Seichim.

I was very unsure of myself and did not feel prepared when I first started teaching Reiki and Seichim. Yet I also knew I had to begin somewhere, and the only way to accomplish this was to "just do it." I developed basic handouts and gradually, the students began to arrive. As I completed each class, I noticed that having to put into words what I had been experiencing as both a practitioner and teacher was a tremendous lesson in itself.

I realized that I understood more than I had been giving myself credit for. I also found that the energy stream itself expanded my capacity for teaching and passing the energy to others, integrating more into my energy system each time I taught a class and gave an attunement. Continuing my ongoing personal healing work also contributed to my growing confidence in my abilities as a teacher.

The same advice found in the previous section beginning on page 86 about Establishing a Healing Practice would apply to becoming a teacher of both SSR and SKHM.

Teaching SKHM

As was previously mentioned, many people today are using the terms Seichim, Seichem, Sekhem and SKHM interchangeably and do not differentiate them. Even Patrick has used different names for the same energy over the years, beginning with Seichem for a very short period and then using Seichim for many years. More recently he has adopted the name SKHM.

Today when Patrick uses the term SKHM, he is referring to both the basic energy stream from which all related healing systems have sprouted as well as to a specific approach he has developed for working with SKHM (as described in the section entitled Patrick

Zeigler's Approach to Healing with SKHM, page 26). As a result of this evolution, not everyone using the term SKHM is necessarily referring to Patrick's approach.

Patrick and the members of the first SKHM teacher's training participated in an intense and accelerated learning process that included developing and designing a curriculum to educate and prepare people as SKHM teachers. Upon successful completion of the entire course, one becomes certified as an SKHM teacher. Patrick's vision is that all who are certified to teach SKHM will do so and will then certify others.

The first group met once a week for a year through telephone conferencing. We also participated in an e-mail list that was made up of only group members. We were together in person three times during the year for two or more days each time. In addition, the format for the group included monthly individual SKHM healing sessions with Patrick.

Members of the group learned techniques for facilitating an individual's healing process both in person and over the telephone as well as methods for helping another person ground the SKHM energy stream. This entailed learning to lead the SKHM Group Attunement Meditation, Healing Attunement Technique and the Infinity Dance found in Appendices V, VI and VII as well as other advanced methods for facilitating and supporting a person through the release, integration and spontaneous initiation process.

We practiced these techniques and methods with each other one-on-one and in the group setting. As well, each member learned how to use these methods to further his or her own personal healing process. We were also encouraged to organize our own SKHM groups and to work with others individually to practice and refine the skills we were learning. These advanced techniques and methods are discussed more throughly in the companion book authored by me entitled *ALL LOVE FOR TEACHERS: A Manual for Teaching Sekhem-Seichim-Reiki and SKHM*.

Working together in these ways with the SKHM energy stream over the course of a full year brought about very profound healing and many positive changes in each group member's life. I have personally come away with a fuller appreciation of the vastness of SKHM and its unlimited capacity to help a person become an open and clear vessel of unconditional love and to let go of anything and everything that is not love. SKHM just keeps on going, and going and going! I also have very much appreciated being on both the giving and receiving ends of the kindness and support the group members gave to each other as the group evolved. In the process, a very deep respect and love for each member of the group developed inside of me, including those who completed the entire year and those who for one reason or another, did not. This love also extends beyond the group to encompass all of creation and life itself. I feel a very soft and warm glow coming from my heart which feels quite wonderful!

This Guidebook also benefitted greatly from my participation in the course in at least three ways. Firstly, the course supported me in healing those issues that stood in the way of my completing the Guidebook which also happened to be the same issues that have kept me from fully standing in my true light and power in other areas of my life. Secondly, I received tremendous inspiration from the group and the heightened SKHM energies that became available through several spontaneous initiations that I received during the year. Thirdly, the course itself provided me with the information about SKHM that was needed for the relevant portions of the Guidebook.

Other group members have voiced similar sentiments. Beverly Oettle expressed her experience of our SKHM course:

> I have found this to be a most incredible year, working with this class and the SKHM energy. This system has helped me reach within myself to heal deep emotional issues and become a clearer channel for healing others. SKHM has given me the ability to give unconditional love, enabling me look past human behaviors to love the soul within. Before starting this class, I suffered from low energy levels, constant stomach pain, and problems with short-term memory to name a few. The energy has given me the skills to overcome emotional and physical barriers on a daily basis, leaving me able to concentrate on lifelong goals I had never dreamed were attainable. I was on a spiritual search when I found Reiki and had studied other energy systems as well. Yet it was the profound self attunement attained through SKHM that enabled me to connect with the Source in a way that continues to spiral and grow each time I work with it.

An instantaneous connection was made with SKHM the moment I found the ad for the SKHM teacher training course. The ad had such an overwhelming effect on me that I cried for two weeks before I was able to make the phone call to Patrick to enroll. The call was equally as passionate as the two prior weeks, with me crying on the phone almost unable to speak, as the breadth of what was to come was already apparent. Now that the class is over, the devotion I have to the SKHM energy will continue to nurture me and everyone that I touch. What began as a one-year commitment to the course has turned into a lifelong dedication to the SKHM energy.

Marsha Nityankari Burack, shared her thoughts about SKHM and our year-long group experience:

I found SKHM to be an emotionally rich, high energy experience. The process encouraged me to safely remember, reexperience and release core wounds on a gut emotional and cellular level. This new and open space was then expanded through meditation, visualization, music and dance. SKHM is truly wonderful!

Another group member, Marie Fouche, wrote the following to describe her experience of the our one-year SKHM class, including a spontaneous initiation that she received:

I will never forget the first day of class. I was very intimidated by everyone else. I felt as if I was a novice attempting to travel intellectually and spiritually further than I could ever hope to move. I listened quietly to everyone as I tried to not hang up the phone and walk away from something I was strongly drawn towards. Patrick began the visualization, and within moments, I embarked on an adventure with SKHM. I instantly felt the vitality of it, chose to take its hand in mine, and LET the SKHM energy show me the way.

I have witnessed incredible healings with SKHM, and I feel so blessed to learn from this energy. Something that the energy tells me to share

with my students all the time, and what I will share with you now, is to remember that the energy is alive! It is not static, nor is it a two-dimensional drawing on a flat piece of paper. It is alive, and it is just waiting for us to interact with it. It is there hoping we will pay attention to it, listen to it and learn from it. The SKHM energy is the true teacher of SKHM. I may teach for another fifty years, and during that time, I will only learn a drop of the infinite possibilities SKHM is capable of. There are no limits to this energy system, or any energy system, except for the limits we impose upon it. Let go of your own limitations, your own fears, and you will see the infinite possibilities. It is amazing how truly infinite love is. Fly with the energy!

Since that first class, I have come to realize the meaning of SKHM for myself. I've been told that SKHM means "Power of Powers," which translated in my personal dictionary means, "Inner Truth." Through the course of this past year, SKHM took me on a journey in search for my Inner Truth. It quickly identified those areas that lacked love and were shrouded within confusion. It helped me dismember those areas where I lied to myself, due to deep fears born many years ago. It let everything fall apart, so I could see what was there all along. I saw many different parts of the whole, and slowly I began the process of rebuilding myself, discovering my true "Essence," and honoring that through being truthful with myself. Doing this has not been easy, and it has not always been joyful. This brought great change into my life, which means I let go of many, many things. However, the end result is really looking good. I am excited about what will come into my life.

Back in February [1999], I went through an initiation experience, which I feel I did not complete until the last day of our year-long course with Patrick. It started off with me going into a deep emotional release regarding a recent and a long ago emotional trauma. At the end of it, I had to lie down. I was exhausted, but I also began feeling a lot of energy trying to move into me. My body began to twitch, and my hands felt so full of energy. I could barely stand it. This is when I saw the infinity swirling above me, and I could feel my energy begin to swirl with it. I felt huge rushes of energy move through me. It was hypnotic, yet I resisted it. I honestly thought there was no way I could physically handle all of that energy. I began twitching more. My feet moved uncontrollably while I shook my hands continuously. I wanted it to stop, but Patrick encouraged me to move through the resistance. I noticed that the more my body moved, the closer the infinity moved to me, and I knew what it was about to do. It was going to merge with me, it wanted me to become one with it. I gave into it, let go of my fear, and it moved into me.

The energy I felt surpasses any possible description I could give to you. However, there was a definite message with it that I wish to share with you as my ultimate lesson from this class, from this energy. As I sat there, I felt all of this love pouring into me, and all I wanted to do was share it with everyone and everything that existed. Within myself, I heard, "I am the Infinity and We Are ALL LOVE." I saw how all of us are love, that is what we are created from, and this physical, very dense body of ours is very good at helping us forget that. I saw that the people we perceive as dark, just have forgotten that love, or have very little love in their lives. They have surrounded themselves with so much hatred, fear and so many other lower emotions, that they have pushed their love deep within themselves, and they can no longer feel it.

It is still there within them, and maybe as someone like that crosses our paths, an opportunity will be before us. I saw how instead of being repulsed or reacting from fear towards a person, I could share this energy with them through a smile, through a kind look, through a loving tone in my voice, or through a gentle touch. By not reacting out of fear, I have the opportunity to share something with them, to help them remember the love that is within them. If I react out of fear towards them, I am being a mirror of their own fears and supporting that behavior within them. Instead, I can choose to respond to them by becoming a mirror of that love within them! "Who knows what kind of flower may bloom from that one moment," I was told.

As I sat there with the energy, "I kept saying, "WE ARE ALL LOVE," and I could not stop crying and laughing at the same time. I realized that my heartbeat was my reminder of how we are ALL LOVE. This truly is a wonderful gift, a beautiful way to look at the world, and hopefully I will be able to walk more peacefully and lovingly upon the Earth Mother and amongst All My Relations because of what the energy shared with me. My heart is with you as you embark upon this journey. We Are ALL LOVE.

Natalie Barton, our group member from "down under," commented about her life and the changes she has gone through as a result of taking the course:

I met Patrick in February 1998 when he visited New Zealand to teach SKHM [then known as Seichim] courses. Having already completed Reiki Mastership and worked with the Tera Mai system, I thought I knew SKHM. Well, that workshop changed my life! I went through the most incredible initiation of my energy career, and things have continued building since. This is one of the things I like about SKHM — you never reach the top, it just keeps expanding.

As I said goodbye to Patrick at the airport in Auckland and walked away I thought, "Wow, imagine working with that guy for a year." Of course, it seemed an impossible dream, until he advertised for the year-long group that I could participate in from anywhere in the world, and did. Coincidence after synchronicity after coincidence occurred, and everything just fell into place.

SKHM has taught me I am always in exactly the right place doing exactly what is needed for my growth, and this course has contributed to that growth considerably. If I thought the first workshop changed my life, think again Nats! During the last year my life has been turned upside down and round about several times, and then jiggled just for fun. The learning that has come about has been quite profound. The energy has supported me throughout the changes (and sometimes not when I have shunned it), yet it is always there in a gentle way when I return. I have discovered more about who I am and what I want and do not want, where I am going, and how to get there in the calmest way possible. And I know that everything is perfect.

Energy equals change, no matter which system you learn, and you can resist or go with the flow. Try both and see the difference! My advice to anyone who cares to listen is—do not be scared and jump in with two feet, and know you must be willing to open your heart and soul to get the fullest benefit. The more you open, the more you receive.

Yes, my life fell apart, and it is being reconstructed beautifully. Cuddles my pussycat agrees as she licks my eyelid while I type this. SKHM, to quote my group members, is truly wonderful, amazingly infinite and a life-long dedication, and I add, "beyond words."

Patrick also shared about his experience of teaching the first SKHM one-year class, as well as the process he and the group went through:

When I began the year-long training it was a first for me. I was working with my inner guidance and the inner voice kept after me until I put out a notice about the class. I thought to myself, "How can I begin a year-long class without an outline or any previous experience teaching using this new format?" Up to that point I had been teaching classes that lasted from two to four days plus my weekly evening class. Now I was looking at the possibility of connecting with people from all over the world once a week on the phone for a year. Yet the voice kept telling me, "trust." I set the class size at twelve and decided that I would not put any filters on who would join so that the first twelve who made a verbal commitment would be part of the first group. This process was absolutely amazing to me because within a couple of weeks the class was full!

The energy of the group was very powerful. Everyone was so excited as we began. When I explained to the group that I had no plan or outline about what would take place over the next year, the energy within the group started to shift. It seemed that some had come to the group with preconceived ideas about how a class should be conducted. It was through many of these issues of structure that fear surfaced in the group. After facing our fears, the greatest lessons of love were received.

I view the one-year course as a cycle of life. Those who finished the course were able to see how important it is to go through the complete cycle of experiencing the SKHM energy as a group for a whole year. Yes, there were some very difficult times that many of us went through over the course of the twelve months. Yet I know for myself this last year has been one of the most transformational periods of my life, and to my surprise and delight the resulting shifts and changes have come from living out fully the true life experiences that were manifested from having created, taught and participated in the course.

I feel so honored to be a part of teaching and sharing SKHM. I want to thank all of the people who were members of the group, including those who did not stay for the entire year. Each of them added his or her unique personal essence to the groundwork that was laid during the first one-year SKHM class. Through our interactions and experiences together, the foundation of what we today *call SKHM has been laid. I especially wish to thank Diane for her labor of love in documenting the class and SKHM in such a beautiful way, and sharing it with the world through her gift of the written word. [Author's note: My pleasure!]*

Future SKHM groups are expected to have a format that may vary from the one described above for the first training group. See the section entitled Contact Information, on page 159, for information on finding a certified teacher of SKHM.

Teaching Sekhem-Seichim-Reiki

SSR is usually taught in a series of workshops that include instruction in healing with SSR as well as other related areas of interest. Each of the classes also includes receiving an attunement from the SSR Master Teacher. This section first discusses Phoenix Summerfield's Seichim system and then provides a basic overview of how the original seven-facet SSR structure came into being, including a description of each of the seven facets. Also included is a discussion of how I have more recently been teaching SSR by combining one or more of the facets into a single attunement and class. There is also a brief discussion of class requirements.

Phoenix Summerfield's Seichim System

The Seichim system developed by Phoenix Summerfield and passed to me included seven facets of Seichim and three of Reiki, with the first three attunements combining Reiki I, II and III and Seichim Facets I, II and III. The final four attunements included Seichim Facets IV, V, VI and VII. At Reiki III (Reiki Master Teacher), the student was able to give attunements for all three degrees of Reiki as well as Seichim I, II and III. At Facet VII (Seichim Master Teacher), the individual learned new information on giving attunements for Facets I through VII.

Although it is clear from Phoenix's teaching literature and paperwork that she used the term "facet," somewhere in my lineage the word "facet" was changed to "level." Until recently, I continued to use

the word "level" as I was originally taught. I have chosen to return to the term "facet," however, because I feel it is a more accurate descriptor for SSR. I see the entire SKHM energy stream as one great universal diamond having an infinite number of facets, with each facet representing the various dimensions and frequency ranges that are available for healing and evolutionary purposes. Use of the term "facet" also helps in eliminating any hierarchical implications of the word "level" which is inappropriate where SSR and SKHM are concerned.

The Original Sekhem-Seichim-Reiki System

Recall that in 1997, I experienced a spontaneous initiation that brought enhancements to the Seichim and Reiki energies I was already working with (see the section entitled The Sekhem-Seichim-Reiki and SKHM Story). At that time, I was inspired to add the third component, Sekhem, including the Sekhem symbol, Heart of the Christos. Initially, I was guided to include seven facets of Sekhem to be transmitted alongside the Seichim and Reiki energies, with the energy flow from the Sekhem symbol being further amplified with each attunement.

What follows is a description of each of the seven attunement facets for the SSR healing system as it was originally structured, including a brief description of the symbols received at each facet (see the section entitled The Sekhem-Seichim-Reiki Sacred Symbols, beginning on page 40, for an in-depth description of the symbols):

SSR Facet I empowers you to channel SSR energy for a lifetime. You receive training in various healing techniques including scanning the auric field, hand positioning on and off the body for treating others and self-healing, angelic light weaving and toning. This attunement opens the lotus blossom of the heart to the Sekhem symbol, Heart of the Christos, activating and stimulating the ongoing process of balancing the physical, emotional, mental and spiritual bodies and unifying all polarities within the various levels of your being. Heart of the Christos is further energized at each successive attunement, which augments and expands the power of this important symbol. Your title after completing this facet is SSR I Practitioner.

SSR Facet II opens you to receive increased SSR living light energy and expands the energy matrix through the teaching of four sacred symbols. The symbols direct the SSR energy for specific uses including releasing energetic patterns held in the physical and subtle bodies that no longer serve the individual, giving mental and emotional treatments for reprogramming the cellular memory, amplifying the amount and degree of energy utilized, and sending SSR healing from a distance. The names of the symbols empowered during this attunement are Cho Ku Rei "A" and "B," Sei He Ki and Hon Sha Ze Sho Nen. After completing this facet, you are an SSR II Practitioner.

SSR Facet III (Reiki Master Teacher) adds two sacred symbols known as Reiki Dai Ko Myo and Seichim Dai Ko Myo. The first is the Reiki Master Teacher symbol. Among its many uses are the opening, balancing and grounding of the central light column to the Earth. Seichim Dai Ko Myo opens the central light column to directly connect with the Source of ALL LOVE. At Facet III, you are taught how to give attunements for passing the SSR energy to others. You may give attunements for SSR Facets I, II and III as well as teach classes in them. Upon completing this facet, you become an SSR III Practitioner and a Reiki Master Teacher.

SSR Facet IV provides a sacred symbol called Cho Ku Ret that works multidimensionally to dissolve barriers to the higher self and the indwelling I Am Presence. This symbol helps to open your capacity to channel and receive information in various sensory forms from spirit guides, teachers, angels, archangels, the ascended masters and the Source of ALL LOVE. It also opens your ability to communicate with plants, animals and the mineral kingdom. In addition, this symbol facilitates being able to access the Akashic records and can be used for empowering objects such as crystals and stones for healing purposes. Upon completing this facet, you are called an SSR IV Practitioner and a Reiki Master Teacher.

SSR Facet V adds a sacred symbol named Shining Everlasting Flower of Enlightenment that dissolves barriers in the emotional body and heart, empowering you to manifest unconditional love and your heart's desires and soul purpose. This symbol also enhances your ability to create prosperity, health and fulfilling personal relationships. You are now an SSR V Practitioner and a Reiki Master Teacher.

SSR Facet VI adds a sacred symbol called Shining Everlasting Living Waters of Ra that is used for releasing deep negative patterns in the physical, emotional, mental and spiritual bodies. It simultaneously purifies, protects, synergizes, integrates and unifies all levels of your being and encourages integration of all polarities such as masculine and feminine. Completion of this facet makes you an SSR VI Practitioner and a Reiki Master Teacher.

SSR Facet VII (SSR Master Teacher) gives the sacred teaching symbol that incorporates all of the other Seichim symbols into one master symbol: Shining Everlasting Living Facets of Eternal Compassionate Wisdom and Healing. The Sekhem symbol, Heart of the Christos, is now fully activated and empowered within you. As an SSR Master Teacher (and a Reiki Master Teacher), you may give attunements for Facets I through VII and teach classes. The attunement process is supplemented to incorporate the entire SSR energy matrix.

The original combined SSR energy matrix included seven facets of attunement for becoming a Sekhem-Seichim Master Teacher and three for becoming a Reiki Master Teacher. The three degrees of Reiki were taught together with the first three facets of Sekhem-Seichim. The attunement sequence varied according to the student's background:

- A student who was already a Reiki Master began by receiving Facets I, II, III and IV of Sekhem-Seichim in one attunement, then received the remaining three facets of Sekhem-Seichim one at a time, for a total of four attunements.

- A student who was a Reiki II practitioner began by receiving Sekhem-Seichim Facets I, II and III and Reiki III, then received the remaining four facets of Sekhem-Seichim one at a time, for a total of five attunements.

- A student who was a Reiki I practitioner began by receiving Sekhem-Seichim I and II and Reiki II. Next the student received Reiki III and Sekhem-Seichim III together, followed by the remaining four facets of Sekhem-Seichim one at a time, for a total of six attunements.

- A beginning student with no previous Reiki training received each facet one at a time for a total of seven attunements.

Recent Developments

Early in 1998, I began to combine facets as I realized that today many people are able to open to and receive greater amounts of the living light SSR energy within a single attunement. This reflects the infinite unfolding process of the SSR and SKHM energy stream. Thus, more recently I have used the following attunement sequence when appropriate for the student:

- For someone who is already a Reiki Master, I have been offering all seven facets of Sekhem-Seichim in either one or two attunements depending on guidance from Spirit.

- A student who is already a Reiki II practitioner receives Sekhem-Seichim Facets I, II and III and Reiki III at the first class, followed by one additional class that combines Sekhem-Seichim IV-VII, for a total of two attunements. (In some cases, I have completed the preceding in just one attunement on guidance from Spirit.)

- A student who is already a Reiki I practitioner first receives Sekhem-Seichim I and II and Reiki II. Next the student receives Reiki III and Sekhem-Seichim III together, followed by one more class that includes Sekhem-Seichim IV through VII, for a total of three attunements.

- A beginning student receives SSR Facets I and II in one attunement, leaving Facet III to be completed separately. The remaining facets are then provided in one or two steps, depending on the individual, for a total of either three or four attunements.

I am currently developing a new curriculum in the form of an in-depth workshop format for teaching the entire SSR healing matrix in two or three days regardless of the student's previous Reiki training. The curriculum will also include aspects of Patrick's approach to healing with SKHM. See the section entitled Classes, Workshops, Speaking Engagements and Healing Sessions with Diane Ruth Shewmaker, on page 159, for more information about SSR attunements and classes.

As an SSR teacher, you will need to decide whether to combine facets when teaching SSR as described above. This is entirely your choice. While I teach Sekhem, Seichim and Reiki together and have been combining facets successfully for some time, others may not feel guided to do the same. I know of some SSR and Seichim Master Teachers who prefer that a student first complete all three degrees of Reiki and then add SSR or Seichim. I also know teachers who continue to teach SSR and Seichim in seven separate steps.

I am frequently asked about the readiness of students to receive more than one facet and/or all three energies at one time. I have found that a teacher's ability to attract students who are ready for such an accelerated path directly correlates with the teacher's belief system and attitudes toward this subject. As you come to a place of peace inside yourself about how to present SSR, people will show up at your door who are ready for whatever you are willing to offer.

Class Requirements

Some master teachers have requirements that must be completed and sometimes documented before a person is eligible to take the class for the next facet and be certified. These requirements can include waiting for a minimum amount of time between classes; receiving a certain number of healings; performing a specified number of in-person and distance healings; reading particular books; writing essays, articles and papers on related topics; practicing attunements; developing a client summary form, a client consent form and a market plan; and setting up classes. You will have to decide what requirements, if any, you wish to have. Ask within about what is appropriate for you and your students.

Sekhem-Seichim-Reiki Practitioner and Master Teacher Attunements

SSR divine light attunements are available to all who desire to connect with this universal energy stream to become a practitioner and master teacher or for personal healing. Each attunement is a heart initiation that further awakens, illuminates and accelerates your soul journey and the divine plan carried within the heart as your soul purpose and blueprint. The result is more love, happiness, joy and peace, which you then extend to others.

Sekhem-Seichim-Reiki Attunement Ceremonies

Center and balance yourself before performing any attunement using whatever methods work best for you, such as prayer, meditation and chanting. I also recommended preparing and clearing the physical space where the attunement will take place. See the sections entitled Preparing Yourself and Preparing the Physical Space, on page 61, for more information.

In the case of a group attunement, I usually place the chairs either in a row with everyone facing the same direction or in a circle facing the center. Take care to leave enough space for you to walk around the entire group as well as sit on the floor to attune the feet. Also, leave enough space between the chairs to allow for angelic light weaving during the attunement.

Before beginning, I remind each person in the group to be receptive to the flow of the attunement process at all times during the ceremony, even when my hands are placed on another person. This avoids any confusion or feelings on a recipient's part of needing to wait for his or her turn.

You will find that the more attunements you give, the more your capacity as a channel of SSR will expand. For example, the first time I worked with three people at once, I was surprised when halfway through the attunement, I began to feel a bit wobbly because of the unusually high energy surges coming through me. I steadied myself, slowed the process down and was able to finish. Soon thereafter, my energy system, including the central light column, adjusted to the increased flow of the energy stream. I was now able to attune four or more people at the same time, though to this day I prefer to work with a maximum of four.

The total attunement time for a single person can last anywhere from twenty-five to forty minutes. When you attune as many as four people at once, the time frame will extend to about an hour for everyone. I recommend you begin by attuning one person at a time to accustom yourself to the process. Then, as you feel ready, add one more person at a time, taking care to not overexert yourself.

If at some point you wish to teach a larger class, you can divide it into smaller groups for attunement purposes. For example, in a class with six people, divide the group in half and complete the ceremony while the other half meditates, studies or takes a meal break. Then do the second small group while the first is engaged in another activity.

When you first begin giving attunements or when you have not performed the ceremony for some time, it is entirely acceptable to keep a copy of the procedure and symbols nearby so you can recover your place quickly if you lose your way. Having the copy close at hand will also help to eliminate any feelings of anxiety over forgetting what comes next or how a given symbol looks.

It is helpful if you can relax and let go of any pressure you may be putting on yourself to do an attunement perfectly and get it all "right." Even if you later realize that you forgot what you consider to be a major step in the attunement, you can follow up by sending it to the person from a distance. Remember too that you have great support and assistance coming from the ascended realms as well as the Source of ALL LOVE.

As you do more attunements and learn to connect each of the steps and phases into one continuous flow, you will find that it becomes easier and more joyful each time. You will also become highly sensitive to the many dynamics that take place during an attunement and will come to know the energetics of each hand position very well.

SSR has two attunement ceremonies for empowering another person as a practitioner and teacher. Either one works well. Though I am now using the second method almost exclusively, I am including both

of them here for historical purposes, as well as to offer the SSR Master Teacher a choice of methods.

The new SSR Master Teacher might initially consider using the first ceremony for a time because its highly repetitive nature will significantly open and widen his or her central light channel as well as strongly assist in his or her continuing integration of the SSR energy stream. These two attunement methods are referred to as SSR Attunement Ceremony "A" and SSR Attunement Ceremony "B."

ATTUNEMENT CEREMONY "A"
AS TAUGHT AT FACET III

Appendix X outlines all of the instructions for performing SSR Attunement Ceremony "A" while this section provides background and explanatory information about these instructions and various aspects of the ceremony. Ceremony "A" is taught to students in two stages. The first stage is detailed in this section and is provided as part of the SSR Facet III class (which includes Reiki Master Teacher). Students in this class learn how to give attunements for SSR Facets I, II and III. This same attunement process is then augmented and strengthened in the second stage at SSR Facet VII so that the new SSR Master Teacher can provide attunements for all seven SSR facets. Ceremony "A" is the same whether you have been attuned to SSR Facet III or SSR Facet VII, with one exception involving the string of beads used at each hand position which is explained in detail in the next section entitled Attunement Ceremony "A" as Supplemented at Facet VII.

SSR Attunement Ceremony "A" is largely based on the attunement procedure passed to me as part of the Seichim system developed by Phoenix Summerfield. After my first weekend experience with Patrick Zeigler, however, I received inner guidance to expand and enhance the ceremony to incorporate the entire SSR healing matrix.

One example of this expansion was to open the central light column at the beginning of the attunement. Another example was to add attuning the feet, which grounds and anchors the SSR matrix more effectively within the receiver and to the center of the Earth. Since many Reiki lineages do not empower the feet, this includes adding language when doing an SSR attunement to attune the feet for those degrees of Reiki that have previously been received by the recipient. See the instructions for attuning the feet in Appendix X for this language.

Though most forms of attunement ceremonies are performed with the student sitting down, I have included directions for the student to either sit in a straight-back chair or lie down on a massage table during the attunement. When I have only one person in a class, I have found that being on a massage table allows for greater comfort and deeper relaxation on the individual's part and is not detrimental to the ceremony in any way.

Ceremony "A" includes three distinct phases:

Phase 1 You will be readying the recipient and opening the sacred space in which the attunement process takes place. There are several self-explanatory steps in this phase that are found in Appendix IX.

Phase 2 You will be attuning the recipient at each of the following positions one at a time in the order listed: (1) the top or crown of the head, (2) the shoulders, (3a) the fingertips, (3b) the palms and backs of the hands, (4) the heart, (5) the third eye and (6) the feet. In each of these hand positions:

- You will first **set your intention that the SSR energies and symbols for the appropriate attunement facets enter each of the positions** and flow through the receiver's physical and subtle bodies in specific ways as detailed below.

- You will next silently **activate and empower the SSR energies and symbols using specific empowerment language** in each of the hand positions. The procedure is the same for each position except for some variations for positions 3a and 3b (fingertips and hands) and position 5 (third eye) as indicated in Appendix X.

- Finally, you will **anchor, seal and stabilize the area being attuned by using the appropriate string of beads** before moving on to the next position. You will use the same string of beads at each hand position.

When you first place your hands in each of the hand positions, allow a few moments to sense and feel the receptivity of the area. Take whatever time is necessary to open and establish the flow of energy in each area. This normally takes no more than a few seconds. During the entire process of activating and empowering each of the areas, set the intention that the energies and symbols will enter the location (including the physical and subtle bodies) as follows:

1. **Crown**—See the thousand-petaled lotus flower of the crown chakra opening and receiving the flow of light from the Source of ALL LOVE in the Great Central Sun. Send the flow down the central light column into the center of the Earth. Ask for the central light column to be widened if you sense this is necessary. Once the central light column is open, send the flow from the column into all of the chakras and sideways throughout the body to establish a gentle opening in the entire energy system of the person.

2. **Shoulders**—See the flow entering the neck, throat and shoulders and traveling through the arms, elbows, wrists, hands and fingers. Also see the flow moving down the neck and throat, through the torso, down the legs and out the feet into the Earth.

3a. **Fingertips**—Move the flow into the tips of the fingers and through the knuckles to the palms of the hands.

3b. **Palms/Back of Hands**—See the energy opening the flow in the palms and back of the hands. Also move the energy through the fingers and wrists as needed.

4. **Heart**—Invoke the Great Central Sun residing in the heart chakra while intending that the SSR energy build and concentrate throughout the chest area. Then expand and radiate the flow of the en-

ergy of the Great Central Sun like a sunburst into all levels of existence while at the same time balancing and unifying these levels within the heart.

5. **Third Eye**—Move the flow into the third eye and into both the pineal and pituitary glands. Then expand the flow throughout the right brain, the left brain and the cerebellum. Also include the balance of the head region including the sinuses, eyes, ears and mouth. When you blow three times into the crown area after completing the string of beads (refer to the instructions for the third eye area in Appendix X), see the energy flowing down the central column and moving wherever it is needed throughout the physical and subtle bodies.

6. **Feet**—After placing your hands on the feet, draw the flow from the upper body down through the legs. Intend for the flow to move throughout both feet taking care to ground and anchor the SSR energy in both feet and the Earth. Also draw the flow from the upper portions of the central light column downward all the way into the center of the Earth and anchor the column there.

You need not memorize every detail of the above descriptions. Rather, simply become clear on the intended flow of the SSR energies at each hand position and use these few moments to be sure each area is open and receptive before proceeding.

The next step in Phase 2 is to use specific empowerment language at every hand position for activating and empowering the SSR energies and symbols. Repeat each phrase silently three times before moving on to the next phrase. When the empowerment language refers to an SSR symbol, you may either (1) draw the symbol above the hand position while saying its name silently to yourself one to three times, or (2) you may invoke the symbol simply by repeating its name silently in your mind while beaming it from one of your palms or your third eye into the position. Choose your method for this according to your level of integration of the symbol per the discussion found in the section entitled The Sekhem-Seichim-Reiki Sacred Symbols beginning on page 40.

The key word in each of the following statements is "empowerment," which together with the SSR Master Teacher's intention and the Will of the Source of ALL LOVE opens the receiver to channeling the SSR energy stream as well as each of the designated symbols. If you use a symbol's name by itself without the word "empowerment," you are invoking its use for healing alone, not for attunement purposes. Where one or more symbols go with the facet, you are empowering that facet simply by empowering its symbol(s). The empowerment language for SSR Facets I, II and III is as follows:

SSR Facet I:
- Reiki I empowerment (3x)
- Seichim I empowerment (3x)
- Heart of the Christos I empowerment (3x)

SSR Facet II:
- Cho Ku Rei "A" and "B" empowerment (3x)
- Sei He Ki empowerment (3x)
- Hon Sha Ze Sho Nen empowerment (3x)
- Seichim II empowerment (3x)
- Heart of the Christos II empowerment (3x)

SSR Facet III:
- Reiki Dai Ko Myo empowerment (3x)
- Seichim Dai Ko Myo empowerment (3x)
- Heart of the Christos III empowerment (3x)

If you are attuning someone who already has Reiki I, II or III, adjust what is to be empowered accordingly by either adding or deleting one or more lines of the empowerment language. Include the symbol Cho Ku Rei "B" for people who have not received it during their prior Reiki II and III training. In addition, some Reiki Masters have not received the SSR version of Reiki Dai Ko Myo. If this is the case, I recommended that you empower the SSR version during the attunement because of its close relationship to Seichim Dai Ko Myo. The following chart clarifies how to attune recipients who are already students of Reiki by listing what needs to be empowered for each SSR facet:

Already Reiki I and moving to SSR Facet II:
- Cho Ku Rei "A" and "B" empowerment (3x)

- Sei He Ki empowerment (3x)
- Hon Sha Ze Sho Nen empowerment (3x)
- Seichim I and II empowerment (3x)
- Heart of the Christos I and II empowerment (3x)

Already Reiki II and moving to SSR Facet III:

- Cho Ku Rei "B" empowerment (if needed) (3x)
- Reiki Dai Ko Myo empowerment (3x)
- Seichim I and II empowerment (3x)
- Seichim Dai Ko Myo empowerment (3x)
- Heart of the Christos I, II and III empowerment (3x)

Already Reiki III and adding SSR Facets I, II and III:

- Cho Ku Rei "B" empowerment (if needed) (3x)
- Reiki Dai Ko Myo empowerment (SSR version) (3x)
- Seichim I and II empowerment (3x)
- Seichim Dai Ko Myo empowerment (3x)
- Heart of the Christos I, II and III empowerment (3x)

The last step in Phase 2 at each of the hand positions is employing the string of beads to anchor, seal and stabilize the area. There is one long and one short version of the string of beads for the SSR Facets I, II and III teacher that are discussed below. Both versions move and anchor the SSR energies and symbols into the physical, emotional, mental and spiritual bodies and through all levels of the central light column, which then opens the unified heart chakra.

The long version is to be worked with until the master teacher has more fully integrated the entire string of beads as discussed in the section entitled Integrating and Working with the Sekhem-Seichim-Reiki Sacred Symbols, on page 54. Though there will be a point at which the master teacher will feel ready to use the short version of the string of beads, I strongly recommend that even then you continue using the long version as often as possible.

One advantage of the long version is that it allows the process to be completed incrementally, one step at a time, providing a longer and sometimes smoother integration period at each of the designated attunement positions. The long version also makes it easier for you to pinpoint those areas of the recipient's energy system that may need greater attention at a later time.

See the section entitled The Human Auric Field, on page 1, for a brief explanation of the various bodies that are sealed and balanced at this stage in the process. The long and the short versions of the string of beads for the teacher attuned through SSR Facet III appears on the next page.

The following example illustrates how the three steps described in the preceeding paragraphs for each hand position in Phase 2 of an attunement combine into one continuous flow. The example uses the heart chakra hand position and assumes the teacher has been attuned through SSR Facet III and is attunung the student to SSR Facet I:

(a) **Place your hands on the front and back of the heart chakra,** establish rapport and set the intention for the flow of SSR energies as described above.

(b) **Voice silently the empowerment langue:**

- Reiki I empowerment, Reiki I empowerment, Reiki I empowerment.
- Seichim I empowerment, Seichim I empowerment, Seichim I empowerment.
- Heart of the Christos I empowerment, Heart of the Christos I empowerment, Heart of the Christos I empowerment.

(c) **Voice silently the string of beads:**

Cho Ku Rei "A"

Cho Ku Rei "B"

Sei He Ki

Hon Sha Ze Sho Nen

Reiki Dai Ko Myo

Seichim Dai Ko Myo

Heart of the Christos

Allow the SSR energies to guide you as to the proper pace and timing so that you are not mechanical while doing an attunement. For one person the pace may be slow and deliberate and for another, more rapid. If you go too fast, often the energy will slow you down by blanking your mind out for a few moments. If you slow down and stay quiet inside, within seconds you will find that the next statement or symbol

Version	String of Beads	Areas Sealed and Balanced
Long	Cho Ku Rei "A"	Physical including etheric
	Cho Ku Rei "B"	Physical including etheric
	Sei He Ki	Emotional
	Hon Sha Ze Sho Nen	Lower mental (concrete mind)
	Reiki Dai Ko Myo	Central light column to heart of the Earth
	Seichim Dai Ko Myo	Central light column to heart of the Source
	Heart of the Christos	All bodies (includes spiritual) + entire central light column + unified heart chakra
Short	Reiki Dai Ko Myo	Physical including etheric + emotional + lower mental + central light column to heart of the Earth
	Seichim Dai Ko Myo	Central light column to heart of the Source
	Heart of the Christos	All bodies (includes spiritual) + entire central light column + unified heart chakra

String of Beads: Long and Short versions for the teacher attuned to SSR Facet III

will easily pop into your mind when it is time to use it.

Timing may also vary between hand positions. I have found this to be particularly true for the heart. At this chakra, I always take whatever time is needed to allow the heart to open up and expand at its own pace with the flow of the SSR energy stream. This can sometimes take several minutes. If it feels necessary, I gently remind the recipient to breathe more deeply, and I rotate the symbol Shining Everlasting Living Facets of Eternal Compassionate Wisdom and Healing through the heart chakra to assist with the opening.

Phase 3 At this stage of the attunement process, you will use angelic light weaving to further move the SSR energies and symbols into the physical and subtle bodies to achieve balance and integration. There are several other self-explanatory steps in Phase 3 detailed in Appendix X that draw the attunement process to a close.

After the attunement is completed, I ask all present to share what took place for them during the attunement if they are willing to do so. I make sure to remind the group that each person's experience will be unique to his or her reference system and the sharing is not intended to be used for comparing one experience to another, which many people are quick to do. Rather, its purpose is to enrich all group members through the awareness of the many different ways an attunement may be experienced. I also suggest that the group write in their journals about what took place. I encourage this sharing and journaling because the grounding and manifestation process is enhanced when a person articulates and/or writes down his or her experience.

ATTUNEMENT CEREMONY "A" AS SUPPLEMENTED AT FACET VII

After completing Facet VII and becoming an SSR Master Teacher, you will be able to attune others for all seven facets of SSR. For Facets I, II and III, the empowerment language is the same as detailed in the previous section. For Facets IV through VII, the empowerment language follows. Repeat each line three times:

SSR Facet IV:
- Cho Ku Ret empowerment (3x)
- Heart of the Christos IV empowerment (3x)

SSR Facet V:
- Shining Everlasting Flower of Enlightenment empowerment (3x)

- Heart of the Christos V empowerment (3x)

SSR Facet VI:

- Shining Everlasting Living Waters of Ra empowerment (3x)

- Heart of the Christos VI empowerment (3x)

SSR Facet VII:

- Shining Everlasting Living Facets of Eternal Compassionate Wisdom and Healing empowerment (3x)

- Heart of the Christos VII empowerment (3x)

At SSR Facet VII, the string of beads expands to include all 11 SSR sacred symbols. The previous string of beads is now replaced with a new long version and two short versions for all attunements. The same discussion found in the previous section concerning how to choose which version of the string of beads also applies for SSR Facet VII. Do not be discouraged from using the long version of the string of beads. As you integrate it within yourself more and more, you will soon find the entire string simply gliding into each of the hand positions with little effort on your part.

Please refer to the section entitled The Human Auric Field on page 1 for a discussion of the various bodies that are sealed and balanced at this stage of the attunement process. The three versions of the string of beads for the teacher attuned through SSR Facet VII are shown in the chart on the next page.

ATTUNEMENT CEREMONY "B"

SSR Attunement Ceremony "B" has unfolded more recently as an outgrowth of the first ceremony, reflecting how the SSR and SKHM energy stream is constantly evolving and finding new ways to be expressed. The ceremony's development was also influenced by my participation in Patrick Zeigler's SKHM teacher's training group which greatly intensified the grounding of the SSR and SKHM energy stream within me. I have been testing this ceremony for over a year and have found it to be much simpler than the first, yet equal to or greater in power than Ceremony "A." Consequently, I now use Ceremony "B" exclusively.

Attunement Ceremony "B" can be found in Appendix X. It is identical to Ceremony "A," with four exceptions. Therefore, the discussion on how to perform an SSR attunement found in the previous section on Ceremony "A" still applies except for these differences, which are explained below.

Phases 1 and 3 are exactly the same, except for one addition at the end of Phase 1. Here are found two of the two primary differences between the "A" and "B" ceremonies. At this point in Ceremony "B," you will be placing your hands on the person's crown chakra while making a statement of intention that includes which SSR facets and symbols are being empowered.

The second difference is to next invite in whatever energy and light transmissions (in addition to those provided as part of the SSR attunement) the person is ready to receive from the Source of ALL LOVE This invitation effectively opens up the potential of the attunement to expand and go beyond what can be thought of as a ceiling or lid that is placed on the person when the attunement template is restricted by language that only includes the particular SSR facet(s) and symbols being empowered.

Although this kind of expansion can also spontaneously take place using Ceremony "A," I have been aware of it more often when using Ceremony "B." A particular kind of light language transmission often occurs that is similar in effect to downloading a computer file. Though I am most often not privy to the full details of the information that is being downloaded, in general it often has to do with the person's soul purpose and activating the next phase of his or her healing process and service work. The person may not always be aware of the transmission at the time it takes place. However, the information will become consciously accessible to him or her when the timing is appropriate.

The third difference is a change in the empowerment language used at each hand position. The earlier version of the empowerment language is replaced with one simple phrase, "ALL LOVE empowerment." You will repeat the phrase "ALL LOVE empowerment"

Version	String of Beads	Areas Sealed and Balanced
Long	Cho Ku Rei "A"	Physical including etheric
	Cho Ku Rei "B"	Physical including etheric
	Sei He Ki	Emotional
	Hon Sha Ze Sho Nen	Lower mental (concrete mind)
	Reiki Dai Ko Myo	Central light column to heart of the Earth
	Seichim Dai Ko Myo	Central light column to heart of the Source
	Cho Ku Ret	Spiritual (higher abstract mind)
	Shining Everlasting Flower of Enlightenment	Spiritual (buddhic)
	Shining Everlasting Living Waters of Ra	Spiritual (atmic)
	Shining Everlasting Living Facets of Eternal Compassionate Wisdom and Healing	Spiritual (monadic)
	Heart of the Christos	All bodies + entire central light column + unified heart chakra
Short#1	Reiki Dai Ko Myo	Physical including etheric + emotional + lower mental + central light column
	Seichim Dai Ko Myo	Central light column
	Shining Everlasting Living Facets of Eternal Compassionate Wisdom and Healing	All levels of Spiritual
	Heart of the Christos	All bodes + entire central light column + unified heart chakra
Short#2	Heart of the Christos	All bodies + entire central light column + unified heart chakra

String of Beads: Long and Short versions for the teacher attuned to SSR Facet VII

at least three times while drawing the flow of the Source of ALL LOVE through you to each of the hand positions, taking whatever amount of time is needed before invoking the string of beads. No longer is it necessary to go through the many lines of empowerment language found in Ceremony "A." The intention statement and the invitation for additional energies made at the crown chakra covers this completely.

The final difference is when attuning the feet. Using additional empowerment language at this hand position for persons who have previously received Reiki I, II and/or III is no longer necessary.

Attunements and the Healing and Purification Process

While the primary purpose of an attunement is to open you to being a channel for the flow of the SSR energy stream, it is also true that attunements greatly accelerate your personal healing and growth. This is because they clear the physical, emotional, mental and spiritual bodies of whatever is in the way of your being an open and loving channel. The discussion found in the section entitled The Heart of Healing, beginning on page 35, explains the healing process and is highly relevant for someone who receives an SSR attunement. Please refer to this section for more information.

When Is It Time for Another Attunement?

There is no prescribed schedule to follow in terms of how much time should pass before a person receives the next attunement. The timing varies from person to person. I rely almost entirely on when the individual's inner guidance and heart say it is time to proceed, as each person knows him or herself best. Rarely have I found that my guidance is different from theirs. When this does occur, either the universe steps in and creates a postponement in the recipient's own schedule, and/or I suggest delaying the attunement. Be assured that all will follow in right timing and right action for those who have chosen this sacred path of illumination and truth.

Oftentimes a person is actually ready for the next attunement, yet has doubts and does not trust his or her feelings of readiness. This arises mainly out of a preconceived notion that every aspect of a given attunement facet must be entirely mastered before having the next attunement. If this were the case, it is unlikely that anyone would ever move beyond his or her first attunement, since one's ability to understand and integrate each of the facets is constantly unfolding. I am still adding to my knowledge of Reiki and expanding my capacity to be a Reiki channel and teacher even though I received my earliest Reiki attunements more than 17 years ago.

Sometimes a person also believes that he or she must be an active SSR practitioner and/or teacher in order to receive the next attunement. This is not al-ways true. Readiness is more about when it is time for that person to receive a greater opening of his or her capacity as a conduit of the energy stream rather than whether or not he or she has opened a practice or taught classes.

Not everyone who receives attunements will feel called to follow the path of becoming a practitioner and teacher. Instead, he or she will carry the SSR energy in whatever way is meaningful for his or her chosen soul journey and purpose. In fact, a person never once has to place his or her hands on another person in order to use SSR for healing, because SSR becomes a part of the person's energy system. Each individual's timing and way of working with SSR is uniquely his or hers and should not be modeled after another person's path.

Distance Attunements

Distance attunements are controversial in some circles. Once you become an SSR Master Teacher, you will have to decide this question for yourself. Some who favor distance attunements feel that if it is possible to send an equally effective healing in person or by distance, then the same is true of attunements. Others disagree with this statement.

Performing distance attunements also brings up the question of how to demonstrate healing methods, communicate the information provided during an in-person class, and observe and guide the progress of the student. Because these considerations are difficult to surmount, many master teachers will not provide distance attunements. I have also heard of some who will do the attunements but will not give certification. Quite a few master teachers, however, are finding success using methods such as teaching on the Internet.

Though I have a strong preference to perform attunements in person, circumstances have arisen where I have been guided to send them from a distance. In these cases, I have found the attunement process equally as effective. However, where possible, I have also followed up with in-person attunements at a later date.

To perform a distance attunement, I prepare the room the same way I would for an in-person ceremony. I use Hon Sha Ze Sho Nen at the beginning, then go through exactly the same steps as an in-person attunement, taking the same amount of time. Depending on my guidance, I either envision the recipient sitting on a chair or lying on my massage table.

Elements of a Sekhem-Seichim-Reiki Class

When teaching SSR, I include a combination of information dissemination, demonstration, practice time and, of course, the attunement itself. I recommend you adopt a format similar to the following example, taking care to include appropriate opportunities for answering questions, sharing of participants' experiences and taking breaks. Set the hours of the class based on the pace at which you are comfortable. Your first several classes may take longer than your later ones, since you likely will find you are able to cover the subject matter in less time as you gain teaching experience:

BEFORE CLASS
❑ Prepare the room and select music.
❑ Prepare yourself.
❑ Complete administrative matters such as preparing class materials, certificates and a roster of students.
❑ Greet students and complete registration, including collecting any amounts due.

INTRODUCTION
❑ Introductions of class members and teacher.
❑ Participants share their answers to the following questions:
  • "What brought you to the class and attracted you to SSR?"
  • "What previous experience do you have with healing, and healing modalities such as Reiki and SSR?
  • How will you be using SSR?"

  • If coming for another attunement, "what have you experienced since the last attunement and how have you been using the SSR energy?"
❑ Provide an overview of the class.
❑ Discuss and answer questions related to SSR in general.

PERFORM THE ATTUNEMENT
❑ Prepare students for the attunement, including a brief introduction to what facets and symbols the students will be receiving.
❑ Perform the attunement.
❑ Take a silent break during which students journal their experiences.
❑ Share attunement experiences with the group, including the teacher's observations.

DISCUSS SSR AND RELATED TOPICS
❑ SSR definition, benefits and overview of the entire SSR system.
❑ The SKHM energy stream and the SKHM Shenu.
❑ History of SSR and other Seichim/SKHM healing systems.
❑ Basics of the human energy system.
❑ Symbols related to the facet(s) being taught and how to draw and use them.
❑ Qualities and values of a practitioner and teacher of SSR.
❑ Opening a healing practice, including professional standards of care, marketing, financial and other legal considerations.

DEMONSTRATION AND PRACTICE

❏ List and demonstrate the main elements of a typical session, including scanning, using intuitive guidance for the hand positions, angelic light weaving and toning.

❏ Lead hands-on practice of healing exercises working with the symbols, angelic lightweaving and toning.

❏ Share practice experiences.

CLOSING

❏ Discuss the healing process and the possible aftereffects of the attunement, including a healing crisis.

❏ Describe the next available attunement and any requirements that need to be completed beforehand.

❏ Award certificates.

If the class includes participants who have had previous attunements, I omit any of the above topics that have been covered in earlier classes. If the class is for SSR Facet III or VII, the format is adjusted to include the following information on teaching and giving attunements:

❏ Becoming a teacher.

❏ Teaching SSR.

❏ Class format and content.

❏ Discussion of the attunement process.

❏ Demonstration of how to perform attunements.

❏ Practice attunements.

Please note that the outlined format detailed above basically includes the topics covered by this Guidebook. If you use this Guidebook as your text, you can refer the student to the appropriate pages of the text for more detailed study. You could also give reading assignments to students to go over certain sections of the Guidebook prior to class.

When I teach a class in which a person is learning SSR for the first time, I like to include a practice exercise in which students pair up, with one person acting as the practitioner and the other as the recipient lying on a massage table. I then ask the "practitioner" students to intuitively find a place on the recipient's body to place their hands. I instruct the practitioners to ask for only Reiki energy to come through, observe their experience of how the energy feels, and share aloud what they have experienced.

While the students keep their hands in place, I next instruct them to ask the Reiki energy to stop flowing and request that only Seichim energy flow, and then observe how it feels and share. We then do the same with the Sekhem energy. I also ask for feedback from the recipients as to how Reiki, Seichim and Sekhem each feel on the receiving end. The partners then trade places and go through the exercise again. When the exercise is completed, I remind the students to work with all three SSR energies at once, noting that the separation of them in the practice exercise has been for learning and demonstration purposes only.

This simple yet powerful exercise provides students with the opportunity to experience the full spectrum of healing frequencies available using SSR as well as compare how the three energies are similar and how they vary. I have noted that students consistently give certain responses to this exercise. Most students, for example, characterize Reiki as a denser and coarser energy, Seichim as finer and more subtle than Reiki, and Sekhem as even more refined than Seichim. Another common statement is that Reiki comes through hot, while Seichim and Sekhem come through on the cooler side. It is only possible to generalize, however, because each person's feedback system is unique to him or her.

Feel free to use your creativity in adding other topics to the class format and developing your own teaching materials. If you wish to use anyone else's materials and information, be sure to obtain appropriate permission and acknowledge the source, even if the material is not copyrighted.

I have included for your convenience the following list of items that I find helpful to have available in my SSR classes:

❑ Roster of students.

❑ Registration information, including amounts due.

❑ Envelope for payments.

❑ Receipt book.

❑ Name tags and marker pen.

❑ CD/tape player and music.

❑ Writing board and pens or chalk.

❑ Class manuals and handouts.

❑ Teaching notes and outline.

❑ Tissues.

❑ Massage tables (I prefer one for every two or three students).

❑ Sheets, pillows, pillow cases and blankets.

❑ Straight-back chairs for attunements.

❑ A crystal bowl, Tibetan bells or other instrument if needed for the optional sound portion of the attunement.

❑ Candles, incense, matches, flowers (and other items as you wish).

❑ Brochures, flyers and business cards.

❑ Water, tea and healthful snacks.

❑ Cups, napkins, utensils.

❑ Certificates and special pen for signing.

❑ Certificate seals.

❑ Embosser for certificate seals.

❑ Paper and pen for recording correct spelling of names for certificates.

Take care in designing your certificates, as your students will very much appreciate your attention to this detail. You can find many distinctive papers available on the market today for your certificates that can be preprinted or used in laser printers. Office supply stores usually carry gold seals. You can also order an embosser for the seal that includes your name and title as an SSR Master Teacher. Below is an example of the certificate that I give to my students.

You may also refer to the companion book, *ALL LOVE FOR TEACHERS: A Manual for Teaching Sekhem-Seichim-Reiki and SKHM*, which provides additional suggestions, further training and class materials for teachers of SSR and SKHM.

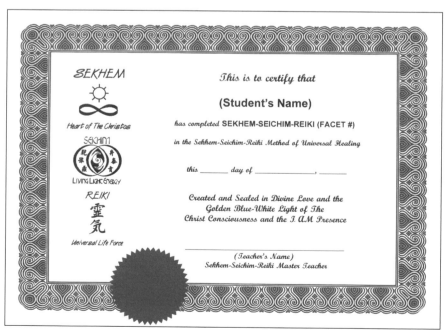

SSR Certificate: The is a sample SSR certificate laser printed on pre-printed certificate paper with a blank gold seal.

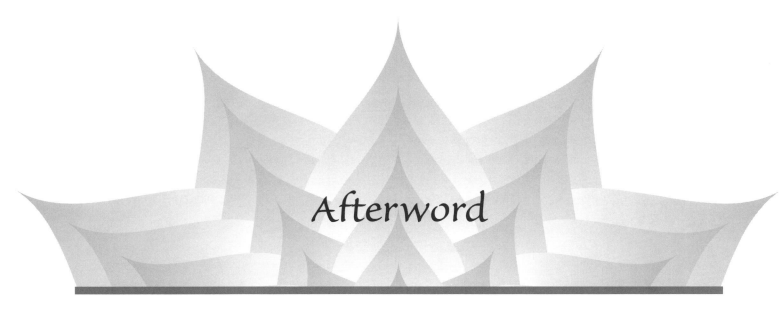

Afterword

Visioning the Future that is Now

Patrick Zeigler was driving home with his daughter through the Virginia countryside the evening of New Year's Day 1999. There was a fine mist hovering in the air that together with the light of the full moon made the landscape appear ethereal and luminescent. Patrick noted that a cross had appeared in the sky formed by two jet streams.

He continued driving and as he watched the sky, he noticed the full moon and the cross begin merging together. It occurred to Patrick that if he were viewing the scene from just the right perspective, the moon and the cross might intersect at the exact center of the cross. To his surprise, as the moon and the cross merged, they instead formed the shape of an ankh.

Patrick called the ankh to his daughter's attention, yet did not think much more about this experience until the next day when he and I spoke on the telephone. He had called me in response to a message I left for him during the afternoon of New Year's Day. In that message, I told him I had just had an exciting breakthrough and insight into the original SKHM shenu design, which he had created some years before and

which we had been conversing about near the end of December.

I told Patrick that during my meditation on New Year's Day, an ankh had appeared to me, visually emerging out of the flower in the shenu as I was contemplating its meaning and design. I also shared how my body had been filled with chills and waves of joy since that moment of discovery. I then pointed out how the ankh was already embedded within the original shenu design.

Patrick then eagerly relayed his New Year's Day ankh experience to me. As he completed telling his story, we both began to vibrate and felt spontaneous initiation energies streaming into our bodies. Even today as I recall this experience, I have chills running up and down my spine and feel like my body is a gigantic smile.

This conversation was an "aha" experience for both of us. We knew our experiences were synchronistic and were indicative that the next phase of grounding the SSR and SKHM energy stream was in full motion. Recall that this energy stream has come back into consciousness in modern times in stages, first with the spiraling energy of Reiki, which was later joined by the infinity flow of Seichim. Now it is time for the next step of more fully grounding and integrating the ankh, or the breath of life, which is the energy of Sekhem and eternal life.

We are taking our first baby steps in crossing over the threshold of a new era in which love and compassion will reign supreme and all of life will at long last come home to abide in the heart of the Source of ALL LOVE. All will join as One in truly living Heaven on Earth. This reality is not as far in the future as some might believe. Many lightworkers have already awakened and are in the process of creating lifestyles that reflect this divine vision and purpose, and are busy helping others do the same. **We are at the dawning of a future that is now.**

The following excerpt from Phoenix Summerfield's literature on Seichim dated February 1988 gives us some insight into her view of this matter in a section called "Spirit in Action":

A subtle, yet compelling shift of focus is affecting our society. Hungering for fulfillment and meaning, people seek the harvest of spiritual food…. Now is the time to claim our power. As we respond to our desires for meaningful lives, we are enabled to respond to one another.

When we choose to balance and heal ourselves, we can experience the dissolution of inappropriate patterns. In action in our lives, we can feel the freedom that comes from releasing negative thoughts and emotions. Character weakness can be replaced with the strength and courage to change our world.

Healed and at peace, we are like pebbles tossed in a pond, affecting all those with whom we come in contact, inexorably and gently, in ever widening circles.

This is a clarion call for unity and cooperation among all lightworkers, including those working directly with the universal SSR and SKHM energy stream, to come together and heal any remaining vestiges of fear, competitiveness and ego within themselves. When this moment of true joining is at hand, another wave of this vast and infinite energy stream will be-

come accessible that we can all share. Truly, there is enough for everyone. Patrick addresses this unity in a 1998 e-mail:

Finally in January 1996 we [Patrick and Phoenix Summerfield] met in Hawaii. I found it quite a coincidence that T'om also showed up at my door several weeks before I left. Because of the timing, it felt as if we were all together…. My feeling was at that time, energetically a shift took place. It was not one person creating a shift but all of us coming together.

Seichim [SKHM] is very much a group oriented energy. I feel it is more holographic in nature than linear. This is why the idea of a lineage bearer does not apply to the energy. Phoenix, T'om and I have never made any such claims. I have used the term founder because it did initially start with me (and it took 12 years for me to use it), but it has been the combination of all who created what SKHM is today. Phoenix, T'om and I were all in agreement on this point. We were also in agreement not to separate the energy.

What is your vision of today and what it could be like? How can you make a difference? What is your sphere of influence? What is your role in creating this vision now in the present moment and making it a lasting reality? Is your vision in alignment with universal law and the highest realms of light? Will your plan be of service to the whole and will it assist everyone in being fulfilled, including you? Are there others who you can join with in sharing a common vision and purpose? How can you create Love and Compassion in Action in every moment of today?

Awaken and activate now the consciousness and power of your heart. Release and let go of all of your fear, unworthiness, doubt, worries and anxiety as well as your feelings of not being ready or adequately prepared. If you are having any difficulty healing yourself, answering any of these questions or putting your vision into action, honestly ask yourself the simple question, *what am I pretending not to know?* Then genuinely listen, accept the truth of what you hear and take action accordingly. Trust that you do have all the answers within your heart because you are ALL LOVE. Wake up and remember. The time is NOW.

In keeping with this call to awaken and remember our true nature and who we really are, I close with a channeled poem titled *The More I Remember…*by Debra Ann White Burch—"Dreamseeker" who is an SSR Master Teacher:

The more I remember –
The more I feel the separateness fall away, and I want to reach out and give to others.
For in that giving, I give to myself, and I feel a part of Everything in Me and Me in Everything.

The more I remember –
The more I see at least a spark of Light in Everyone.
I can no longer look for the darkness, but rather, through love and compassion,
I see the Light grow and shine like the brightest star in each and Everyone.

The more I remember –
The more I hear only truths touching my ears.
Untruths are only fleeting illusions and carry no real substance,
While truths are like music to my ears and to which my whole body resonates and dances with joy.

The more I remember –
The more I find myself talking to the animals, insects, trees, rocks, stars and seas, and I find they talk to me.
Their simple, yet wondrous ways spark my memories and they thank me because I listened -
    I Listen.

The more I remember –
The more I can taste the sweet taste of life itself.
We all came from the same place and we are all going to the same place.
Life is that journey,
And there is no sweeter taste than being fully present in the here and now.

The more I remember –
The more I take the time to "smell the roses."
I learn to appreciate each flower my journey brings me.
Yes, even the weeds have beauty and a unique scent.
By slowing down, I can see all of the details in each life event more clearly.

The more I remember –
The more I truly know and understand myself and realize –
I am not alone – no, not ever – NEVER.
For I am at one with myself and in that

I am One with All – ALWAYS – ALL WAYS.

Ω
Omega
Benediction

You have now arrived at what appears to be an ending. Even so, nothing is further from the truth. Instead, now is the time and place for action and for you to rededicate yourself and begin anew, fully rejuvenated, restored and uplifted in body, emotions, mind and spirit as well as in purpose.

Because SSR and SKHM flow from the universal Source of ALL LOVE, like the Source they represent totality and oneness as well as the unity of All That Is, including all space, all time and all spirit. They are the Alpha and the Omega, the beginning *and* the end. Likewise, you hold the Alpha and the Omega within your heart and soul. Within this infinite space lies One Truth. One Voice. One Breath. One Mind. One Spirit. One Heart. One Love.

Be fully secure in the knowledge of your purpose as a divine vessel of the Universal Love, Wisdom and Power that ceaselessly radiates from the Source of ALL LOVE. Know that your path clearly has been laid before you. No longer need you harbor in the hidden recesses of your heart any fear or doubt as to who you really are or why you have chosen to be on the planet Earth at this time in Her evolution. You are here to give ALL LOVE. You are here to receive ALL LOVE. You are here to be ALL LOVE. You are here to teach ALL LOVE. You are here to take action in alignment with ALL LOVE. In truth, you are ALL LOVE.

ALL LOVE. ALL LOVE. ALL LOVE. ALL LOVE. ALL LOVE. ALL LOVE. ALL LOVE. ALL LOVE. ALL LOVE. ALL LOVE.

Mother Mary, Queen of Heaven
Channeled through Diane Ruth Shewmaker

Appendix I: Invocation to the Unified Chakra

I breathe in Light
Through the center of my heart,
Opening my heart
Into a beautiful ball of Light,
Allowing myself to expand.

I breathe in Light
Through the center of my heart,
Allowing the Light to expand,
Encompassing my throat chakra
And my solar plexus chakra
In one unified field of Light
Within, through, and around my body.

I breathe in Light
Through the center of my heart,
Allowing the Light to expand,
Encompassing my brow chakra
And my navel chakra
In one unified field of Light
Within, through, and around my body.

I breathe in Light
Through the center of my heart,
Allowing the Light to expand,
Encompassing my crown chakra
And my base chakra
In one unified field of Light
Within, through, and around my body.

I breathe in Light
Through the center of my heart,
Allowing the Light to expand,
Encompassing my Alpha chakra
(Eight inches above my head)
And my Omega chakra
(Eight inches below my spine)
In one unified field of Light
Within, through, and around my body.
I allow the Wave of Metatron
To move between these two points.
I AM a unity of Light.

I breathe in Light
Through the center of my heart,
Allowing the Light to expand,
Encompassing my eighth chakra
(Above my head)
And my upper thighs
In one unified field of Light
Within, through, and around my body.
I allow my emotional body to merge
With my physical body.
I AM a unity of Light.

I breathe in Light
Through the center of my heart,
Allowing the Light to expand,
Encompassing my ninth chakra
(Above my head)
And my lower thighs
In one unified field of Light
Within, through, and around my body.
I allow my mental body to merge
With my physical body.
I AM a unity of Light.

I breathe in Light
Through the center of my heart,
Allowing the Light to expand,
Encompassing my tenth chakra
(Above my head)
And to my knees
In one unified field of Light
Within, through, and around my body.
I allow my spiritual body to merge
With my physical body,
Forming the unified field.
I AM a unity of Light.

(continued next page)

I breathe in Light
Through the center of my heart,
Allowing the Light to expand,
Encompassing my eleventh chakra
(Above my head)
And my upper calves
In one unified field of Light
Within, through, and around my body.
I allow the Oversoul to merge
With the unified field.
I AM a unity of Light.

I breathe in Light
Through the center of my heart,
Allowing the Light to expand,
Encompassing my twelfth chakra
(Above my head)
And my lower calves
In one unified field of Light
Within, through, and around my body.
I allow the Christ Oversoul to merge
With the unified field.
I AM a unity of Light.

I breathe in Light
Through the center of my heart,
Allowing the Light to expand,
Encompassing my thirteenth chakra
(Above my head)
And my feet
In one unified field of Light
Within, through, and around my body.
I allow the I AM Oversoul to merge
With the unified field.
I AM a unity of Light.

I breathe in Light
Through the center of my heart,
Allowing the Light to expand,
Encompassing my fourteenth chakra
(Above my head)
And to below my feet
In one unified field of Light
Within, through, and around my body.
I allow the Source's Presence to move
Throughout the unified field.
I AM a unity of Light.

I breathe in Light
Through the center of my heart.
I ask that
The highest level of my Spirit
Radiate forth
From the center of my heart,
Filling this unified field completely.
I radiate forth throughout this day.
I AM a unity of Spirit.

Ground multidimensionally. Imagine a thick line of Light beginning at the Omega chakra (eight inches below your spine), extending upwards into the upper part of the unified field. Ground into the vastness of your Spirit. Allow your Spirit to stabilize you. Run twelve lines of light downward from the point of the Omega chakra, opening around your feet like a cone. You are not grounding into the Earth. You are stabilizing yourself across the parallel realities of the planetary hologram.

FROM: *What Is Lightbody?*, Archangel Ariel channeled by Tashira Tachi-ren. Gratefully used with permission.

Appendix II : Sekhem-Seichim-Reiki and Seichim/SKHM Chronology

What follows is a general chronology and summary of the development and evolution of SSR and Seichim/SKHM in modern times. Some of the dates are close approximations as it was not possible to be more exact. The approximations are noted with an asterisk (*). As well, because this time line is in summary form, it is suggested that the reader consult the section entitled The Sekhem-Seichim-Reiki and SKHM Story, beginning on page 11, for the full details.

Late 1800's	Dr. Mikao Usui seeks to learn the method used by Jesus for healing. After many years of searching, Reiki and its symbols are revealed to him during a mountaintop experience. While traveling, he does healing work and teaches Reiki to others.
1925	Dr. Usui initiates Chujiro Hayashi as a Reiki Master. Hayashi opens a Reiki clinic in Japan.
1935	Hawayo Takata is hospitalized in Japan for surgery and learns of Hayashi's Reiki clinic. She opts for treatment at the clinic and in four months is healed.
1936-1937	Hayashi teaches Takata Reiki I and II.
1938	Takata is initiated as a Reiki Master by Hayashi. Soon thereafter, she returns to her native Hawaii and opens a Reiki clinic. She eventually carries Reiki to Europe, Canada and the United States.
1970-1980	Takata trains 22 Reiki Masters before her death in 1980.
1979	Patrick Zeigler's Great Pyramid spontaneous initiation takes place during an overnight stay in the Pyramid.
1979	Zeigler spends two to three weeks with a Sufi group in Egypt and with their spiritual teacher, Sheikh Mohammed Osman Brahani in the Sudan. He learns many spiritual practices, including a Sufi form of dance called "zikir" and the mantra, ALL LOVE.
1979	Zeigler returns from Egypt to Yemen where he is on assignment with the Peace Corps. He begins working with the teachings and practices learned while in Egypt and the Sudan.
Mid-1980*	Zeigler's assignment is moved to Nepal. He continues working with the teachings and practices.
1982-1983	Diane Ruth Shewmaker learns Reiki I and II. She begins having spontaneous initiation experiences.
1983	Zeigler returns to the United States, attends the New Mexico Academy of Healing Arts and becomes a massage therapist. He learns Reiki I and II.
March 1984	Zeigler completes Reiki IIIa. He also returns to the Sudan for a short visit with the Sufi group and learns that the Sheikh has died. The group encourages Zeigler to teach what he learned from the Sheikh.
Summer 1984	Zeigler moves to California and begins teaching and taking classes at a school of massage named Heartwood.
1984	Zeigler meets Christine Gerber who channeled Marat, a 2,500 year-old-spirit guide who was a Seichim teacher in India. Marat tells Zeigler the energy he is working with is called Seichim. Marat gives him other information about Seichim, including the symbol, Cho Ku Ret. Zeigler begins to practice giving attunements for Seichim.
1984	Zeigler meets Tom Seaman at Heartwood and gives Seaman attunements for Seichim, including Reiki III and the symbol Cho Ku Ret.

1984	Zeigler gives Seichim attunements to David Quigley and also studies with him for nine months learning techniques for past life regression and deep emotional process work. Zeigler also assisted Quigley in teaching some classes. This was the formative stage of what later emerged as Zeigler's approach to healing with SKHM.
1984-1985	Seaman begins teaching Seichim. One of his first two students is Faun Parliman who becomes a Seichim teacher.
1985	Parliman meets Phoenix Summerfield (then going by her birth name of Kathleen J. McMaster) in Los Angeles and gives Summerfield her first Seichim attunement, including Reiki III.
1985	Summerfield studies with Seaman and completes her Seichim training. She and Seaman also work together for a short period of time, which included some development work on symbols.
1985-1987	Summerfield creates a seven-facet Seichim system, including adding additional symbols, and begins teaching Seichim at expos and health fairs.
1985 forward	Two distinct styles of teaching Seichim emerge reflecting Seaman's and Summerfield's approaches to working with the energy. As others receive Seichim attunements and become teachers, additional related Seichim healing systems are also created.
1985	Zeigler leaves the United States to live and work in the Sudan for a year.
1986	Zeigler returns to the United States and completes a two-year masters degree in architecture.
1986-1990	Zeigler teaches three Seichim classes while in school. His individual healing work is done chiefly with family and friends. Zeigler chooses to remain in the background of the growing public interest in Seichim as a healing modality.
1987	Zeigler and Summerfield talk for the first time on the telephone. Summerfield sends Zeigler a packet of information describing the seven-facet Seichim system she has developed, including artwork.
1990	Zeigler reopens his healing practice to clients and begins teaching regular Seichim classes again.
1990	Seaman enters a decade-long period in which he spends most of his time with his family.
1991	Summerfield and Marsha Nityankari Burack meet for the first time and become friends.
1992-1993	A series of events in Burack's life leads her to an inner understanding that the Egyptian goddess, Sekhmet, is the guardian of the Seichim energy. Burack introduces Sekhmet to Summerfield and Summerfield incorporates Sekhmet into her Seichim teachings.
1992-1993*	Summerfield begins teaching Seichim in Australia. Seichim spreads throughout the world.
1994-1995	Zeigler studies with Robert Jaffe and Brian Grattan. These studies give Zeigler additional training in techniques for working with others in a group setting and individually.
1995 forward	Zeigler begins to teach more Seichim groups, incorporating the information and skills he learned in his studies with Quigley, Jaffe and Grattan. Zeigler's current approach to healing with Seichim/SKHM more fully emerges.
1995	Burack's book, *Reiki: Healing Yourself & Others* is published, including some of the earliest published information about Seichim.
1995	Shewmaker becomes a Reiki Master and receives her first Seichim attunements from a seven-facet Seichim system developed by Summerfield. Shewmaker begins teaching all three degrees of Reiki and Seichim Facets I-III and reopens a private healing practice.
January 1996	Zeigler and Summerfield meet for the first time in person in Hawaii. Just a few weeks before this, Patrick had been with Seaman. Because of the timing, Patrick felt as if they were all together and that this joining created an energetic shift.

1996	Shewmaker becomes a Seichim Master. Her classes include Reiki and all seven facets of Seichim.
1996	Zeigler is inspired to design the original SKHM Shenu.
June 1997	Shewmaker meets Zeigler at a Seichim workshop taught by Zeigler. Following a spontaneous initiation, she begins to channel another aspect of the SKHM energy stream which she is guided to call "Sekhem." Out of this new understanding, she is led to create a healing system that she names Sekhem-Seichim-Reiki (SSR). Within a month, she incorporates SSR into her teaching curriculum.
Late 1997	Zeigler and Summerfield speak for the last time.
1998	Zeigler discovers the meaning and significance of the last piece of information given to him in 1984 by Marat about the ankh, or breath of life, and incorporates this information into his classes.
1998	Amy Roland's book, *Traditional Reiki for Our Times*, is published with information about Seichim.
1998	Zeigler adopts the name SKHM, instead of Seichim.
Summer 1998	Death of Summerfield.
July 1998	Shewmaker receives additional Reiki Master attunements, including for traditional and Tibetan Reiki.
August 1998	Zeigler begins the first SKHM teacher's training group. Shewmaker and Burack are among its members.
Early 1999	The original SKHM Shenu is enhanced to reflect an expanded understanding of the nature of the SKHM energy stream and its related healing systems.
1999	Seaman's family responsibilities end and he reemerges into the larger community.
August 1999	Seaman and Shewmaker meet for the first time in person. Zeigler and Shewmaker also meet Burack for the first time in person.
August 1999	The first SKHM teacher's training group is completed during the period of the solar eclipse and the grand cross. The group met together for one year.
November 1999	This Guidebook is released and introduces the new version of the SKHM Shenu. It represents the first known in-depth published work that describes the evolution of Seichim/SKHM in modern times as well as a related healing system known as Sekhem-Seichim-Reiki (SSR). The writing of a soon to be released companion manual for teachers is completed.
2000	The New Millennium begins.

Appendix III: Usui Shiki Ryoho Reiki Family Tree of Diane Ruth Shewmaker[1]

SPIRIT

DR. MIKAO USUI

CHUJIRO HAYASHI

HAWAYO TAKATA

JOHN GRAY	IRIS ISHIKURA	PHYLLIS FURUMOTO	BARBARA RAY
Diane Ruth Shewmaker	Arthur Robertson	Pat Jack	Patrick Zeigler[2]
(1982 and 1983)	Karen Cameron	Carol Farmer	Tom Seaman[3]
	Karen Fox	Leah Smith	Faun Parliman[4]
	Marie Ciociolla	William Rand	Phoenix Summerfield[5]
	John Purdy, Jr		Daverna Shields Gabriel
	Randy Clark		Kay Hudson Wohl
	Andrea Arden		Sandra Koppe
	Diane Ruth Shewmaker		Liliana Kilgallen Shenk
	(1998)		Diane Ruth Shewmaker
			(1995)

---

[1] Diane Ruth Shewmaker received Reiki I and II from John Gray and Reiki Master training through the other lineages in the years shown. John Gray is one of the original 22 Reiki Masters trained by Mrs. Takata.

[2] Patrick Zeigler received Reiki I and II from Marilyn Alvy, whose Reiki lineage is not known. He received Reiki IIIa from Barbara Ray prior to her developing The Radiance Technique. Ray is one of the 22 Reiki Masters trained by Mrs. Takata. The lineage shown in this column was named "Seichim" and began when Patrick Zeigler combined the Reiki and Seichim energies and passed them to Tom Seaman, including all of the Reiki symbols and the Seichim symbol, Cho Ku Ret.

[3] Tom Seaman received Reiki I from Phyllis Furumoto and Reiki II from Bethel Phaigh. They both were among the 22 Reiki Masters trained by Mrs. Takata.

[4] Faun Parliman received Reiki I, II and III as part of the Seichim lineage from Tom Seaman. She had not received any other Reiki training at the time she passed the energy to Phoenix Summerfield. Faun later added additional Reiki training.

[5] Phoenix Summerfield received Reiki III as part of her Seichim training from both Faun Parliman and Tom Seaman. Though Phoenix was already a Reiki II, it is not known who she received this training from or if she completed any further Reiki training after studying with Faun and T'om. Phoenix's birth name was Kathleen J. McMaster.

Appendix IV: Sekhem-Seichim Family Tree of Diane Ruth Shewmaker

Sekhem

Spirit

Great Pyramid Experience • Sheikh Mohammed Osman Brahani • Marat

Patrick Zeigler

Diane Ruth Shewmaker

(1997)

Seichim

Spirit

Great Pyramid Experience • Sheikh Mohammed Osman Brahani • Marat

Patrick Zeigler

Tom Seaman

Faun Parliman

Phoenix Summerfield

Daverna Shields Gabriel

Kay Hudson Wohl

Sandra Koppe

Liliana Kilgallen Shenk

Diane Ruth Shewmaker

(1995-1996)

Appendix V: SKHM Group Attunement Meditation

Note to the Reader: This SKHM Group Attunement Meditation is one of the methods used by Patrick Zeigler in the SKHM groups that he leads. While the meditation can be done while sitting quietly, the energy often inspires a more active experience involving body movement and sound such as toning. The meditation also can stimulate a deep release and healing process that is usually completed in the group following the meditation with the support and assistance of the group leader and members of the group. This may then be followed by one or more spontaneous initiations. Refer to the section entitled Patrick Zeigler's Approach to Healing with SKHM, beginning on page 26, for more information in this regard.

Please note that this SKHM Group Attunement Meditation has been included to provide the reader with a method for connecting with the SKHM energy stream as a tool for personal healing. Although the reader is encouraged to experiment with this meditation and hopefully will have a beneficial experience, Patrick has found that it is strongest and most effective when led by an individual who has actively worked with the SKHM energy stream for at least one year.

This greatly increases a person's likelihood of having had a spontaneous initiation experience, which deeply grounds the energy stream into him or her. This grounding, in turn, greatly enhances the person's ability to assist others in activating the SKHM energy stream within themselves. As well, the person will have gained a greater understanding of the SKHM energy stream and how to use it for healing purposes during the course of a year.

Patrick also feels strongly that a person desiring to teach SKHM in a group setting as discussed in the section entitled Patrick Zeigler's Approach to Healing with SKHM must first develop many advanced skills for working with the energy stream both personally and with others. This requires study, practice, support and integration time of at least one year in a framework such as the one-year SKHM teacher's training course (see the section entitled Teaching SKHM, on page 91. for more information on this course). Thus, this SKHM Group Attunement Meditation is intended to be used by the reader for individual healing purposes only. The reader is also referred to the companion volume to this Guidebook entitled *ALL LOVE FOR TEACHERS: A Manual for Teaching Sekhem-Seichim-Reiki and SKHM* for a full discussion of such advanced skills and methods.

❧

Close your eyes and be aware of yourself sitting in our circle. Take a moment to observe and feel a connection with everyone in the circle. Take several deep breaths in and out and feel what is going on within your body. Notice any tension or lightness. If any part of your body feels tight and tense, breathe into that area. Allow it to soften and relax. Feel your breathing going all the way down to your lower abdomen and expanding into the upper part of your chest.

Now bring your awareness to your heart center and breathe into your heart. With every breath in and out, feel your heart expanding. Allow yourself to feel all the sensations within your heart center. Do not judge the sensations; just observe and allow yourself to feel them. If you do not feel anything, then allow yourself to experience the numbness. As you continue to breathe in and out, let your heart expand even more.

Visualize a beautiful flower bud opening right at the crown of your head. Feel a connection between the top of your head and your throat. Within this connection, allow a stem to form that drops down from the flower bud and into the heart. Allow your heart to become a sacred vessel to receive the flower stem. The ancient Egyptian hieroglyph that represents the heart is a vessel with two handles on each side. Visualize that symbol of a vessel with perhaps a beautiful design. Fill the vessel of your heart with your breath and awareness, allowing it to expand and become larger.

Above the top of your head, visualize a brilliant, radiant sun shining its rays down on the flower bud. Breathe the light of the sun through the flower petals, and as they begin to open, receive the light. Breathe it in. Breathe it down into the heart, and as you do, allow the stem to expand and open even more, creating a connection between the top of your head and your heart. Feel the rays of light from the sun shining down into your heart center.

As you breathe in the light of the sun through the flower bud and the stem, a wider column of light coming down from the sun begins to form. Breathe this column open and bring it down into the heart and the belly. Now breathe the column into the base of the spine, through the root center, down through the legs and into the soles of your feet. Feel your feet planted firmly on the ground and imagine that they have roots growing deep into the Earth.

Move the light column down deep into the Earth as well, feeling your connection to the heart center of the planet and anchoring the column there. As you make the connection with the heart center of the Earth, breathe the light of the Earth up through the column into your body. Allow yourself to remember why you are here on the planet. Let those memories begin to surface and breathe into them. If you wish, you can make a commitment to fully be here now on this planet. This does not mean you will be here for an eternity, but just for now, being here fully in all of your essence, in all of your light.

Ask at this time for all of your soul essence to come into your body, inviting it to flow into your heart center, then bringing it all the way down into the heart of the Earth. Feel your heart connecting to the planetary heart. As the Earth begins to receive your light and your presence, feel an exchange of energies taking place between your light and the light of the planet.

Begin to receive the Earth, drawing its light up through your roots and into the soles of your feet. Continue bringing the light up through your legs, then into the base of the spine. Move it into the belly, through the solar plexus, then into the vessel of the heart. Feel the energy of the Earth mixing with the light from Heaven. Feel Heaven and Earth residing in the heart as One.

As the energies of Heaven and Earth merge in the heart center and expand, allow a horizontal energy flow to begin, moving out from your heart and through your shoulders, arms and hands. When combined with the vertical light column running through your body, this horizontal flow forms a cross.

Now breathe the sun above your head down through the column so it rests atop the crossbar in the center of the cross, forming an ankh. Feel your heart receiving the solar disk and the ankh pattern as they merge with your body. Let the ankh be completely integrated within your cells. Let the horizontal flow of light moving through your arms and hands extend out in both directions to the other people in the circle. Send the horizontal energies out into the world and feel all hearts connected as One.

Now be aware of a point several inches above the top of your head and a point several inches below your feet in the Earth. See an egg being formed around you that includes these two points at the top and bottom. The egg completely encircles you and encompasses the Source of ALL LOVE and Heaven and Earth as a unified whole. Feel yourself being held safe and fully protected within this sacred and holy space.

Growing and radiating out from the perimeter of the egg are the petals of the lotus flower of the heart. Feel how your energy system is no longer divided into individual and separate chakras. They are now completely unified. One Heart. One Love. ALL LOVE. Sit inside the space of the unified heart chakra and feel your connection with the Source of ALL LOVE. Hold that space and radiate it out to all of creation. ALL LOVE. ALL LOVE. ALL LOVE.

Now imagine a giant column of light in the center of the circle. While each of us has our own column, we also are able to form this group column of light. Imagine the light coming straight from the Source of ALL LOVE originating at a point far above us and going deep down into the center of the Earth. Visualize those two points above and below the entire group.

Imagine now that at these same two points above and below you are the apexes of two pyramids, one pointing upward and one pointing downward. Feel the shape of the two pyramids coming together to form an octahedron that encompasses our entire circle.

See the pyramids rotating in a clockwise motion. Breathe into the octahedron and feel helixes of light coming into you in a clockwise rotation spinning the octahedron that we are all inside. Allow the spinning to slow down and stop. Now see the pyramids moving in a counterclockwise motion so that the octahedron is spinning in the opposite direction. Once again, feel the helixes of light coming into you.

Now allow the octahedron to spin both clockwise and counterclockwise at the same time. Let the two rotational patterns come together and form an infinity or figure-eight pattern far above the top of your head. Bring the symbol down into the group light column in the center of the circle. Imagine that the column has group chakras running along its length that correspond to our own, and as we work with the group chakras, we are also working on our own.

Bring the infinity pattern down to the crown chakra, letting the pattern form petals of light with each movement. Move the pattern down into the third eye, bringing forth the visualization of the infinity pattern. Move your awareness down to the throat, and in the throat chakra, begin to give the energy you are experiencing a voice—ALL LOVE, ALL LOVE, ALL LOVE, ALL LOVE. Let the voice resonate inwardly. Move the infinity pattern

into the heart, integrating the voice with the expression of love in the heart. Feel the love in your own heart. As you move the infinity pattern through the heart, expand the petals formed by the infinity pattern outward.

Move your awareness down into the solar plexus and bring the infinity pattern into the fire of the solar plexus. Bring forth its power and combine it with the love as One. Breathe into the chakra and feel this power and love, bringing them into unity each time the energy moves to the center point of the infinity pattern. Now bring your awareness down into the second chakra, feeling the inner child. Surround the child with the infinity pattern so that he or she is bathed and soothed in the flow of the energy. Feel a connection to the other people in your life and allow all relationships to be healed.

Move your awareness down to the base of your spine and open the gates of the Earth. With each movement, feel the first chakra opening and receiving the infinity. Allow the root center to spin with the flow of the infinity, then move the pattern down your legs into the heart of the Earth. Feel the infinity below you and breathe into it.

Now breathe the infinity up through your legs and the base of the spine into the second chakra, then up to the solar plexus and into the heart. Allow the pattern to expand into your heart and feel that all of our hearts are connected. Experience each of us as being a petal of a large lotus flower. Feel the infinity moving between us and building a network of light. Breathe into that network.

Feel the ALL LOVE within your heart—ALL LOVE, ALL LOVE, ALL LOVE. Allow the movement to become more delicate as it opens into the stillness of the heart, always there and always present. Slowly feel your connection with each person in the group become even stronger. As you maintain this connection, move into your throat center and let the energy flow through the throat in the form of toning and sound.

(In a group setting, this SKHM Group Attunement Meditation is followed by group toning and process as discussed in the Note to the Reader above and the section entitled Patrick Zeigler's Approach to Healing with SKHM. This moves the group process to a more advanced level.)

Appendix VI: SKHM Healing Attunement Technique

Note to the Reader: This SKHM Healing Attunement Technique is one of the methods used by Patrick Zeigler in the SKHM groups that he leads. The healing attunement can stimulate a deep release and healing process that is usually completed in the group following the activity with the support and assistance of the group leader and members of the group. This may then be followed by one or more spontaneous initiations. Refer to the section entitled Patrick Zeigler's Approach to Healing with SKHM, beginning on page 26, for more information in this regard.

Please note that this SKHM Healing Attunement Technique has been included to provide the reader with a method for connecting with the SKHM energy stream as a tool for personal healing. Although the reader is encouraged to experiment with this technique and hopefully will have a beneficial experience, Patrick has found that it is strongest and most effective when performed by an individual who has actively worked with the SKHM energy stream for at least one year.

This greatly increases a person's likelihood of having had a spontaneous initiation experience, which deeply grounds the energy stream into him or her. This grounding, in turn, greatly enhances the person's ability to assist others in activating the SKHM energy stream within themselves. As well, the person will have gained a greater understanding of the SKHM energy stream and how to use it for healing purposes during the course of a year.

Patrick also feels strongly that a person desiring to teach SKHM in a group setting as discussed in the section entitled Patrick Zeigler's Approach to Healing with SKHM must first develop many advanced skills for working with the energy stream both personally and with others. This requires study, practice, support and integration time of at least one year in a framework such as the SKHM teacher's training course (see the section entitled Teaching SKHM, on page 91, for more information on this course). Thus, this SKHM Healing Attunement Technique is intended to be used by the reader for individual healing purposes only. The reader is also referred to the companion volume to this Guidebook entitled *ALL LOVE FOR TEACHERS: A Manual for Teaching Sekhem-Seichim-Reiki and SKHM* for a full discussion of such advanced skills and methods.

To receive this healing attunement, the recipient may be standing, sitting in a straight-back chair or lying down on a massage table depending on his or her preference. The healer stands. The instructions below are for the healer, including directions to be said aloud to the recipient during the healing attunement. You are encouraged to put the instructions into your own words when giving a healing attunement.

Healer: To prepare yourself to give the healing attunement, close your eyes and come into your heart by focusing your awareness on your heart center and taking a few deep breaths. Feel your heart expanding. Set the intention within yourself for the healing attunement to take place. From the heart, move your attention to the top of your head and open your crown center. Then form your light column by visualizing a brilliant sun above the top of your head. See the sun radiating a column of light that shines over you as well as down through you, filling your heart center, moving down through your spine and traveling all the way into the center of the Earth. Feel connected to the Source of ALL LOVE above you and to Mother Earth below.

Healer: Gently place your hands on the recipient's shoulders. You are going to speak to him or her. It is important to use your voice. As you speak, the energy will move more strongly through your heart and throat centers. While the person is breathing in and out, synchronize your breath with his or her breath. Say:

Take a few deep breaths in and out and close your eyes. Move the breath down into the belly. Let the light of the breath fill the belly and then move it up into the heart and into the chest.

Healer: Stand to the side of the recipient. Take one hand and gently touch the recipient on the upper part of his or her chest in the center. Place your other hand on his or her back directly behind the heart (if the recipient is lying down, slide your other hand under the back behind the heart). By doing this, you are supporting the heart and giving the person some focus. Say:

Bring all of your awareness into your heart by directing your breath in and out of your heart. Feel all of the sensations there. Create a heart chamber—a vessel within the heart. Feel all of the smaller chambers within the heart. Imagine those doors opening up as you breathe the light into those spaces.

Healer: Move your awareness to the top of the recipient's head. Bring your hands up and imagine that you are supporting a beautiful flower bud directly above his or her head. Say:

See a beautiful flower bud above your crown center. Allow the bud to begin to open and breathe in through the flower down into the heart.

Healer: Hold your hands up around the sun and support it above the recipient's head while imagining it radiating down on the person. Say:

Above the top of your head visualize a brilliant sun—a solar disk. Feel the sun radiating down and going into your heart, filling the heart with each breath. Breathe it down all the way into the heart.

Healer: Stand in front of the person. Move your hands in front of the recipient to form a column start-

ing at the level of the sun and motioning down into the center of the Earth. Say:

As the sun radiates down on you, allow it to form a column of light that moves into your heart, your solar plexus, your second chakra and into your base chakra. Visualize the column moving down your legs, through your feet and into the Earth.

Healer: Get down on your knees in front of the recipient and put your hands on his or her feet. Imagine you are anchoring the column in the heart of the Earth. Say:

See the column going deep into the Earth, connecting your heart with the heart of the planet. Let yourself remember why you are here on the planet Earth. If you wish, you may make a commitment to fully be here now on this planet. Feel your heart and breathe in all of your light, all of your soul essence, all of your love—inviting it all into the center of the Earth. Feel the Earth receiving it. Make the connection, and begin to breathe the Earth's light up through the column. Breathe it into your feet and up your legs.

Healer: Move your arms and hands up in front of the recipient's body to support the Earth energy flowing up through the column to the heart. Say:

Keep drawing the energy of the Earth up through the column, breathing it into the base of the spine, the second chakra, the third chakra and into the heart chamber. Also feel the Heaven energy radiating down from the sun and bring Heaven and Earth together in your heart center.

Healer: Without touching the person's body, move your hands horizontally from the center of his or her heart straight across the shoulders and along the arms to form the horizontal portion of the cross. Gently touch the person's hands in the center of each palm while imagining the palm chakras opening up. Say:

As the heart chamber fills, allow the unified flow of Heaven and Earth to move out from your heart through the shoulders and arms and into your hands, creating a horizontal bar that together with the light column forms a cross.

Healer: Reach your arms up to the sun and guide it down through the recipient's crown chakra, bringing it to rest on the center of the horizontal bar of the cross to form the ankh. Say:

Breathe the radiant sun from above the top of your head in through your crown chakra. Bring the solar disk to rest on the center of the horizontal bar of the cross just above the heart center and form an ankh. Breathe in and out and merge that ankh into the physical body. Allow yourself to fully embody the ankh.

Healer: Open the person's right hand so that the palm is facing up. Hold your non-dominant hand under the person's hand. Use your dominant hand to draw a spiral over the palm. Move the spiral into the person's hand by momentarily touching your palm to his or her palm. Next follow the same procedure first with the infinity and then with the ankh. After completing all three symbols, gently release the right hand and repeat the process with the person's left hand. Say:

I am now placing a spiral into the palm of your right hand ... and now I am placing an infinity there ... and now an ankh. [Change to the left hand.] I am now placing a spiral into the palm of your left hand ... and now I am placing an infinity there ... and now an ankh.

Healer: Picture your column of light supporting the recipient's column. Step back and let the person be completely in his or her own space. The person can now be standing, sitting or lying down, as he or she prefers, to integrate the energies. If necessary, gently assist the person with changing body positions. Encourage him or her to be totally relaxed. Say:

You may now be physically standing so that you form the column with your body or, if you prefer, you may sit or lie down for the balance of the attunement. Relax completely and keep breathing. Feel the light inside of you radiating forth from deep within your chest.

Healer: Now begin to work at each chakra with the infinity pattern. Bring your awareness to the person's crown chakra to start. Move your hand(s) over the crown chakra in an infinity pattern. See it rotating around like a flower. Let your body move with your hand motions. This is a meditation for you as well, allowing you to both give and receive a more concentrated flow. You can spend as long as you want at each location. Be comfortable with what you are doing. Say:

I am now going to move the infinity flow through your entire energy system, beginning with the crown chakra. Breathe in and out and allow yourself to open up and receive the flow inside this chakra. As I move to each new area, I will let you know where I am focusing.

Healer: Move down to the recipient's third eye and draw the infinity pattern over this chakra. Do the same for the chakras at the throat, heart, solar plexus, sacral area and base of the spine. Move the infinity to the recipient's knees, feet and into the center of the Earth. Then bring it back up through the feet, legs and knees. Continue moving the infinity through the base, second, and solar plexus chakras, and up into the heart. See the pattern expanding out from the heart. Say:

I am now at the third eye...the throat chakra ...the heart...the solar plexus...the second chakra ...the base chakra...the knees...the feet...and the center of the Earth. The infinity flow is coming back up now through the feet...the legs...and back up through all of the chakras [name them one at a time]. The infinity is now at your heart. Feel the infinity flow expanding your heart and beginning to form the petals of a lotus flower.

Healer: Move one hand to a point several inches above the top of the recipient's head to symbolize Heaven. Do the same with a point several inches below the person's feet to symbolize Earth. Draw an oval in the air around the person to enclose him or her in the cosmic egg as found in the SKHM Shenu. Draw the petals of the lotus flower around the egg. Say:

Now be aware of a point several inches above the top of your head and a point several inches below your feet in the Earth. See an egg being formed around you that includes these two points at the top and bottom. The egg completely encircles you and encompasses the Source of ALL LOVE and Heaven and Earth as a unified whole. Feel yourself being held safe and fully protected within this sacred and holy space.

Growing and radiating out from the perimeter of the egg are the petals of the lotus flower of the heart. Feel how your energy system is no longer divided into individual and separate chakras. They are now completely unified. One Heart. One Love. ALL LOVE. Sit inside the space of the unified heart chakra and feel your connection with the Source of ALL LOVE. Hold that space and radiate it out to all of creation. ALL LOVE. ALL LOVE. ALL LOVE. As you hold that space of ALL LOVE within yourself, move into your throat center and let the energy flow through the throat in the form of toning and sound.

(In a group setting, this SKHM Healing Attunement Technique is followed by group toning and process as discussed in the Note to the Reader above and the section entitled Patrick Zeigler's Approach to Healing with SKHM, beginning on page 26. This moves the group process to a more advanced level.)

Appendix VII: SKHM Infinity Dance

Note to the Reader: This SKHM Infinity Dance is one of the methods used by Patrick Zeigler in the SKHM groups that he leads. The dance can stimulate a deep release and healing process that is usually completed in the group following the activity with the support and assistance of the group leader and members of the group. This may then be followed by one or more spontaneous initiations. Refer to the section entitled Patrick Zeigler's Approach to Healing with SKHM, beginning on page 26, for more information in this regard.

Please note that this SKHM Infinity Dance has been included to provide the reader with a method for connecting with the SKHM energy stream as a tool for personal healing. Although the reader is encouraged to experiment with this dance and hopefully will have a beneficial experience, Patrick has found that it is strongest and most effective when led by an individual who has actively worked with the SKHM energy stream for at least one year.

This greatly increases a person's likelihood of having had a spontaneous initiation experience, which deeply grounds the energy stream into him or her. This grounding, in turn, greatly enhances the person's ability to assist others in activating the SKHM energy stream within themselves. As well, the person will have gained a greater understanding of the SKHM energy stream and how to use it for healing purposes during the course of a year.

Patrick also feels strongly that a person desiring to teach SKHM in a group setting as discussed in the section entitled Patrick Zeigler's Approach to Healing with SKHM must first develop many advanced skills for working with the energy stream both personally and with others. This requires study, practice, support and integration time of at least one year in a framework such as the SKHM teacher's training course (see the section entitled Teaching SKHM, on page 91, for more information

on this course). Thus, this SKHM Infinity Dance is intended to be used by the reader for individual healing purposes only. The reader is also referred to the companion volume to this Guidebook entitled *ALL LOVE FOR TEACHERS: A Manual for Teaching Sekhem-Seichim-Reiki and SKHM* for a full discussion of such advanced skills and methods.

Choose a place ahead of time where you can lie down after the dance. Have a pillow and blanket available in case you need them. You may do this dance to music. Throughout the dance, stand and move or sway your body both physically and energetically in a gentle figure eight or infinity pattern—whichever feels appropriate. Intuitively decide what rhythm is good for you. You can do this dance with your eyes open or closed, opening and closing them at different times according to your preference.

Stand with your feet about shoulder width apart. Take a few deep breaths and bring your awareness above the top of your head. Visualize a brilliant star far above your head and mentally draw a figure eight or infinity pattern coming down from that point. Allow the top of your head to move, drawing the infinity with the motion of your head. Let the energy of the infinity pattern expand. Allow the head to move so that the eyes are looking up and around. This infinity is not two-dimensional; it is a three-dimensional pattern similar to a roller coaster. Feel the roller coaster curves and the movement of the infinity going up, down and around.

As you let the infinity flow and expand out, bring it right to the top of your head. Visualize the infinity forming the petals of the lotus flower of the crown chakra. Feel your crown opening as each petal is formed. Keep breathing into the unfolding, letting the movement take your body over as the crown opens.

Move the infinity pattern into the third eye. Feel the pattern inside the third eye. As the infinity moves throughout this chakra, allow it to open up even more.

Bring the infinity pattern down into the throat and express the words "ALL LOVE" aloud, generating the sound from the throat center. When speaking the word "ALL," bring the tip of the tongue to the roof of the mouth and say, "ALLLLL LOVE, ALLLLL LOVE." Repeat this several times. Feel the infinity pattern and the mantra vibrating in the throat and opening the throat center. Begin to synchronize the mantra with your breath—breathe in ALL LOVE, breathe out ALL LOVE. Let the in and the out breaths vibrate the heart and feel the ALL LOVE deep within your heart center.

Now move the infinity into the center of the heart, feeling the ALL LOVE vibration even more deeply. Allow the infinity to open and expand your heart center. Next bring the infinity down into the solar plexus, feeling the fire in this area and letting the breath move into it. Move the infinity down further into the sacral chakra and embrace your inner child. Bring the love vibration you are generating to that child. Also connect with the other relationships in your life, and allow the ALL LOVE to heal them as well as any sexual trauma lodged within the sacral area. Keep chanting the mantra ALL LOVE aloud or silently within yourself. Bring the infinity down into the root chakra and feel the pattern there, opening this chakra even more.

Feel the foundation of the Earth under you, supporting you and taking care of all your needs. Take the ALL LOVE down into your knees and feel the infinity flowing around them. Bring it deep down into your feet and feel the pattern all around them as well. Now go deep, deep, deep into the Earth, connecting your heart with the heart of the planet. Continue chanting ALL LOVE out loud or silently within yourself.

Begin to bring the infinity flow from the center of the Earth back up through the feet and knees. Bring that light from the Earth up through the base chakra and into the pelvis, then into the belly and up to the solar plexus. Now move it into the heart, ALL LOVE, ALL LOVE, ALL LOVE. Bring the light of the infinity flow into the heart and feel it radiating out from the center, then horizontally through the shoulders, down the arms and out through the hands.

Let your body movements and swaying gradually slow down. Gently stop moving your body and stand still. Take a moment and become very quiet, feeling the energy moving through your body. Slowly, find your pillow and blanket and lie down. As you lie there with your eyes closed, feel the expansion of the energy within you. Experience the movement of the pulsations going through your energy system. Quietly breathe into it. Feel your heart. Feel the ALL LOVE. Notice everything you are feeling. With intention, use your breathing to move the vibration into every cell of your body. Take a few deep breaths.

As you lie there, imagine you are standing with your feet on the Earth. Be aware of a point several inches above the top of your head and a point several inches below your feet in the Earth. See an egg being formed around you that includes these two points at the top and bottom. The egg completely encircles you and encompasses the Source of ALL LOVE and Heaven and Earth as a unified whole. Feel yourself being held safe and fully protected within this sacred and holy space.

Growing and radiating out from the perimeter of the egg are the petals of the lotus flower of the heart. Feel how your energy system is no longer divided into individual and separate chakras. They are now completely unified. One Heart. One Love. ALL LOVE. Sit inside the space of the unified heart chakra and feel your connection with the Source of ALL LOVE. Hold that space and radiate it out to all of creation. ALL LOVE. ALL LOVE. ALL LOVE. As you hold that space of ALL LOVE within yourself, move into your throat center and let the energy flow through the throat in the form of toning and sound.

(In a group setting, this SKHM Infinity Dance is followed by group toning and process as discussed in the Note to the Reader above and the section entitled Patrick Zeigler's Approach to Healing with SKHM, on page 26. This moves the group process to a more advanced level.)

Appendix VIII: Sample Sekhem-Seichim-Reiki Client Consent Form

Note to the Reader: This Sample Sekhem-Seichim-Reiki Client Consent Form is based on information presented in the section entitled Professional Standards of Care, on page 86, which contains a general discussion of this topic. The reader should revise this form to reflect the laws of the state where the healing practice is located and according to his or her individual circumstances.

❧

Welcome to my healing practice. My name is (fill in practitioner's name) and I am a practitioner of a healing system called Sekhem-Seichim-Reiki or SSR for short.

What is SSR?

SSR is a healing system that works holistically to aid in balancing and harmonizing all aspects of a person's being which includes the physical, mental, emotional and spiritual levels of his or her energy field. The positive effects of SSR are cumulative and will carry forward from session to session, building momentum as an individual moves through the healing process.

SSR helps to activate a person's innate healing resources to support healing of acute and chronic disease as well as anxiety, depression, fatigue, and stress. Other reported benefits include improved health, more joy and love of living, increased energy and vitality, enhanced creativity, deeper relaxation, stress relief, increased mental clarity, improved relationships, and a new and powerful recognition of the recipient's unique selfhood. SSR can also assist a person in finding his or her soul purpose, and in enhancing communication with his or her spirit guides, angels, the ascended masters and the Source of ALL LOVE.

SSR compliments and enhances traditional medical interventions. It is not medical or psychological treatment and is not a substitute for such care. As such, you should continue any treatments you are receiving from other health care professionals while you are working with me. There are also no guarantees of a cure or the form in which healing may take place.

The SSR Session

During the energy work portion of your SSR session, you will lie on the massage table fully clothed. I will be gently placing my hands both on and above your physical body. In this way, the SSR energy will be able to access your entire energy field, including all of its levels. I will be using sacred symbols, sound, and angelic light weaving to focus the SSR energies to better facilitate healing. I will be working in partnership with your conscious intent, Higher Self, angelic guides, and the Universal Mind so that the amount of energy received and integrated during your SSR session will be that which best serves your highest good at that moment in time.

During the session you may feel sensations such as tingling, temperature changes, shifts in the breathing rhythm, lightheadedness and vibration. You might have feelings of overall relaxation, peace, joy and love. You may also experience the release of emotions such as anger and sadness, along with the need to cry. This includes remembering experiences from this or other lifetimes that are ready to be cleared.

The Healing and Purification Process

Much of the release experience is relatively gentle, does not take a great deal of time to work through your system and passes almost without notice. Sometimes, however, the manifestations of the clearing process are more noticeable and uncomfortable and may take several hours, days or even weeks to work their way through your energy system. This can be especially true if you are not fully and consciously ready for and accepting of whatever may be changing in your life and can stimulate what is known as a "healing crisis."

As toxins and old ways of being are released from all levels of your being, you may experience one or more of the following symptoms of the purification process: The physical body may have flu-like symptoms, fever, headache, sore throat, coughing, aching joints and muscles, tingling sensations, nausea, constipation and/or diarrhea. Temporary changes may also take place in your sleep habits such as needing to sleep more often and longer and/or being wide awake when you normally sleep. **If you have any severe or continuing physical or emotional reactions or complications after receiving an SSR treatment, please report them immediately to me and to your health care providers. I am not a licensed psychotherapist, psychiatrist, or counselor, and therefore will be happy to refer you to qualified therapists for the processing of any new awarenesses as they surface.**

In all cases, nurture and treat yourself with the utmost love and compassion when going through any form of healing crisis and the accompanying detoxification process. Gently exercise or do yoga. Eat health-supporting foods and drink lots of pure water. Set aside time for yourself and go for walks in nature. Breathe fresh air deeply into your lungs. Relax in water. Sit close to a blazing fire. Get plenty of rest and be very kind to yourself.

You also will find it highly beneficial to surround yourself with a caring support system and take advantage of the many healing modalities that can assist you, including SSR. Both complementary and traditional approaches to your healing process may be appropriate if called for, including herbal remedies, chiropractic treatments, massage therapy, acupuncture, homeopathy, sound therapy, rebirthing, aromatherapy, flower essences, medicines, surgery and psychotherapy. Be sure to allow sufficient time for integration of the SSR process no matter what combination of approaches you choose to use.

Sometimes it is also helpful in clearing toxins to take a cleansing bath before and/or after a session using sea salt, Epsom salts, baking soda or peroxide (the peroxide is highly diluted so it will not cause bleaching of the hair). You can also place a few drops of a favorite essential oil in the bath water. When the bath is complete, take a shower as normal. After drying off, place moisturizing lotion on the body. If you can only take a shower, an alternative is to make a paste of the sea salt, Epsom salts or baking soda and rub the paste on the body, including the chakra areas. When rinsing, request through clear intention that the shower clear the auric field as well.

Number and Frequency of Sessions

The number and frequency of sessions will vary depending on your needs and your goals for our work together. Sometimes only one or a few sessions are all that is required. If you wish to do some concentrated healing work or are in the middle of a crisis period in your life, more frequent sessions spaced one week apart may be of benefit. In other circumstances, the time between sessions may be two to three weeks or even a month. You know yourself and your needs better than anyone else. I will also periodically make recommendations to you about this based on the progress of our work together.

Session Follow-up

Please feel free to call me for any reason after a session should the need arise. I especially want to know about any adverse or unexpected reactions that you may experience so that appropriate action may be taken. Sometimes it is helpful in times like this to do some distance healing as well as to talk by telephone. It may also be appropriate for you to consult with medical or psychological professionals.

Additional Information on SSR as a Healing Modality

For more information about SSR as a complementary healing modality, it is suggested that you read the book, *ALL LOVE: A Guidebook for Healing with Sekhem-Seichim-Reiki and SKHM*, by Diane Ruth Shewmaker. You may order the book from me or from the publisher at: Celestial Wellspring Publications, 6107 SW Murray Boulevard, PMB213, Beaverton, Oregon 97008-4467, 800-966-5857, 503-469-9292, fax: 503-469-9393, e-mail: awakener@celestialwellspring.com, website: www.celestialwellspring.com.

Administrative Policies

My administrative policies with regard to length of sessions, fees and fee structure, cancellations, late arrival and returned checks are as follows:

- **Length of Sessions:** Regular in-person SSR sessions are_____in length. Extended SSR sessions are in length. Distance SSR sessions are usually anywhere between 30 and 60 minutes and are charged by the minute.

- **Fees and Fee Structure:** Payment for services is due at the time of the session unless previous arrangements have been made. My fee structure is as follows:

Regular In-person SSR Sessions:	$_____
Extended In-person SSR Sessions:	$_____
Follow-up Telephone conversations lasting more than 10 minutes:	Prorated
Distance SSR Sessions	$_____/minute

- **Cancellation:** 24-hour notice is required for cancellation of appointments or a $ cancellation fee applies. Missed or forgotten appointments will be charged the full session fee.

- **Late Arrival:** It may not be possible to receive a full session if you arrive late for an appointment. However, the fee for a full session will be due.

- **Returned Checks:** There will be a $_____ charge for any returned checks.

Client Consent

I, (name of client), have read all of the information contained in this Client Consent Form and understand it fully. I acknowledge that it is my responsibility to inform (name of SSR practitioner) and to contact my health care professionals if there are any adverse or unexpected reactions to my SSR session(s). I also understand that SSR complements many modalities of treatment and is not a substitute for medical and psychological treatment, and does not guarantee a cure or the form in which healing may take place.

I further understand I am not receiving medical or psychological treatment from (name of SSR practitioner) and that I should continue to follow the recommendations of my other health care providers while working with (name of SSR practitioner). I also understand and agree to the policies discussed above.

Date:_____ Signed:_____

Appendix IX: Sample Sekhem-Seichim-Reiki Client Summary Form

Note to the Reader: This Sample Sekhem-Seichim-Reiki Client Summary Form is based on information presented in the section entitled Professional Standards of Care, on page 86, which contains a general discussion of this topic. The reader should revise this form to reflect the laws of the state where the healing practice is located and according to his or her individual circumstances.

৯১

Name: _____ (W)Phone: _____

Address: _____ (H)Phone: _____

City/State/Zip: _____ Fax: _____

E-mail: _____ Birthdate: _____

Date of ❏ Visit ❏ Telephone Conversation ❏ Distance Healing: _____

Reason for ❏ Visit ❏ Telephone Conversation ❏ Distance Healing: _____

_____

_____

Background Information Including Previous Experience with Energy Work: _____

_____

_____

Services Provided: _____

_____

Session Notes: _____

_____

_____

Response of Client: _____

_____

_____

Recommendations Made: _____

_____

Date of Next Appointment: _____

Follow-up: _____

Appendix X: Sekhem-Seichim-Reiki Attunement Ceremony "A"

Note to Master Teacher: An explanation for the basic foundation of this attunement ceremony can be found in the sections entitled Attunement Ceremony "A" as Taught at Facet III and Attunement Ceremony "A" as Supplemented at Facet VII.

If you are attuning more than one person at a time, all parts of Phase 1 are completed for everyone together as a group. Walk around everyone in one large counterclockwise circle for the last part of Phase 1. In Phase 2, move from one person to the next and complete each person's crown chakra. Do the same with each person's shoulders, hands and so on until you finish the last position at the feet. In Phase 3, perform the angelic light weaving for each person one at a time. Make the four thumps on the floor and the four claps above your head individually. Then complete the balance of Phase 3 with everyone together as a group.

꒰

Phase 1

1. **Have the recipient sit in an upright chair with his or her hands placed palms up on the lap, or lie down on a massage table with arms placed comfortably at the sides.** Be sure the person has taken off his or her watch, glasses and shoes. If desired, play soft music in the background.

If the person is seated, explain that at a certain point in the attunement, you will be moving and gently slapping his or her hands in a particular sequence ending with the hands being placed on the heart (see Positions 3a and 3b). Briefly demonstrate how you will be doing this. Ask the person to keep the hands in this position for the balance of the attunement, if possible. If not, ask the person to gently place the hands back on the lap with palms up.

Explain that the ceremony is a time of silence, receiving and initiation. Suggest that he or she let go of all preconceptions and ideas of what is about to take place and relax, allowing the experience to unfold in the moment. Ask the recipient to close his or her eyes and keep them closed until completion of the ceremony.

2. **Open the central light column.** Ask the person to breathe more deeply and slowly than normal, breathing in up from the lungs, through the shoulders and to the top of the head, then breathing out all the way down to the bottom of the feet. Suggest that the individual do this several times, making the inhaling and exhaling equal in length and creating a circular flow of energy around the entire body.

After the person has begun to relax and quiet down, if the person is seated suggest that he or she become aware of the central light column that connects the chakras and runs parallel to the spine through the middle of the body, from the top of the head to the base of the spine. (If the person is on a massage table, his or her awareness should be brought to the column running vertically from the top of the head to the bottom of the feet.) Ask the person to open and expand the column by gently breathing in and out several times.

Next ask the recipient to visualize his or her feet standing firmly on the Earth while sending the light column down like roots from a tree all the way into the heart of the planet, anchoring it there. Then ask the person to also extend the column above the head all the way through the celestial realms up to the heart of the Source of ALL LOVE, anchoring it there.

As the person maintains the same breathing rhythm, ask him or her to simultaneously breathe the grounding and supportive Earth energies into the column from below and the celestial Heaven energies into the column from above, allowing Heaven and Earth to come together within the heart region. Here the energies blend, merge, balance and unify as One, filling the heart to capacity.

Encourage the person to allow the unified energies to spill over into the entire circulatory system of the physical body, nourishing all the tissues, organs, muscles, bones and cells. Then have the person expand the flow from the heart like a sunburst into the etheric, emotional, mental and spiritual bodies that surround and interpenetrate the physical body.

Once the initial flow through the central light column has been established, the person does not have to concentrate on the breathing and should be encouraged to allow his or her thoughts, feelings and sensations to move wherever the process takes him or her.

3.   **Soul mantra:** Stand in front of the person (if seated) or at the head of the table (if on a massage table) and with your arms raised in the air, recite the soul mantra aloud three times. Go through the entire verse before beginning again:

> We are the Soul.
> We are the Monad.
> We are the Light Divine.
> We are Love.
> We are Will.
> We are Perfect Design.

4.   **Standing in the same position and speaking aloud, invoke the presence and participation of the angels, guides and teachers of the initiate and yourself as well as the ascended masters and the Source of ALL LOVE.** Invoke them generally or call in certain ones specifically as intuitively guided. Suggest that the initiate silently call in any others he or she wishes to be present.

5.   **Standing in the same position, aloud or silently say:**

> *Thank you. Thank you. Thank you, Holy Father God and Mother Goddess for the privilege of giving this empowerment.*

6.   **Starting from where you have been standing, move eight times counterclockwise around the recipient.** Count on your fingers if necessary to keep your place. Hold your palms in the air, facing them toward the recipient as you walk. Say silently:

> *You, [initiate's name], are free to accept or reject this Sekhem-Seichim-Reiki empowerment. Sekhem-Seichim-Reiki is a harmonizing, healing, balancing and loving universal energy of the Christ Consciousness and the I AM Presence. I ask the healing god Thoth and the goddess Isis to make every moment of this attunement equal to millions of years of healing, wholing and loving.*

Phase 2

1.   **Position 1 - Top of Head:** Stand in back of the recipient with your hands on top of his or her head, fingers together. Draw SSR energy from the Source of ALL LOVE and send it through your hands into the head. As this is taking place:

- Intend the flow of energies and appropriate symbols.
- Silently use appropriate empowerment language (three times for each line).
- Silently use the long or short version of the appropriate string of beads.

2.   **Position 2 - Shoulders:** Stand in back of the person with your hands on his or her shoulders, fingers together. Draw SSR energy from the Source of ALL LOVE and send it through your hands into the shoulders. As this is taking place:

- Intend the flow of energies and appropriate symbols.
- Silently use appropriate empowerment language (three times for each line).

- Silently use the long or short version of the appropriate string of beads.

3. Position 3a - Fingertips (if seated): Stand in front of the person and silently guide the recipient to hold his or her hands in front of the heart in prayer position, with the fingers and thumbs together. Place one of your hands around his or her wrists. Cup your other hand over the person's fingertips and thumbs. Draw SSR energy from the Source of ALL LOVE and send it through your hands into the recipient's finger tips and thumbs. As this is taking place:

- Intend the flow of energies and appropriate symbols.
- Silently use appropriate empowerment language (three times for each line).
- *For this position only, you do not need to use the string of beads, as this is completed for the entire hand area with Position 3b.*

Position 3a - Fingertips (if on a massage table): Stand to the left side of the person and place one of your hands around his or her wrist. Cup your other hand over the person's fingertips and thumb. Draw SSR energy from the Source of ALL LOVE and send it through your hands into the recipient's fingertips and thumb. As this is taking place:

- Intend the flow of energies and appropriate symbols.
- Silently use appropriate empowerment language (three times for each line).
- *For this position only, you do not have to use the string of beads, as this is completed for the entire hand area with Position 3b.*

Now complete Position 3b below for the left hand and then move to the right side of the person and complete Position 3a for the right hand per the above. Then go on to Position 3b for the right hand.

4. Position 3b - Palms and Back of Hands (if seated): While still standing in front of the recipient,

move his or hands so that they are held comfortably side by side, cupped with the palms open and at waist height. Hold the palm of your non-dominant hand under the person's two open and cupped hands so that your palm is placed behind and up against the back of the person's hands. Draw SSR energy from the Source of ALL LOVE and send it through your hand into the back of the recipient's hands. Simultaneously, send SSR energy from the Source of ALL LOVE through your third eye into the person's palms. As this is taking place:

- Intend the flow of energies and appropriate symbols.
- Silently use appropriate empowerment language (three times for each line).
- Silently use the long or short version of the appropriate string of beads.
- *Blow on the cupped palms three times.*

Gently place one of the person's palms over the heart chakra. Take the other open palm and place your non-dominant hand underneath it to support the next motion. Using your dominant hand, flatten out the person's open palm. Then gently but firmly slap the open hand, holding your slapping hand flat on his or her palm for a few seconds before beginning again. Slap the palm a total of three times. Then reverse the person's hands and follow the same procedure. When you are finished with the person's second hand, place it across the other one, over the heart.

Position 3b - Palms and Back of Hands (if on a massage table): While still standing to the left side of the recipient, gently move his or her left hand so that it is open with the palm up. Hold the palm of your non-dominant hand under the person's open hand so that your palm is placed behind and up against the back of the person's hand. Draw SSR energy from the Source of ALL LOVE and send it through your hand into the back of the recipient's hand. Simultaneously, send SSR energy from the Source of ALL LOVE through your third eye into the person's left palm. As this is taking place:

- Intend the flow of energies and appropriate symbols.

- Silently use appropriate empowerment language (three times for each line).
- Silently use the long or short version of the appropriate string of beads.
- *Blow on the cupped palm three times.*

After completing Position 3b for the left hand, move to the right side of the person and complete Position 3a for the right hand. Then come back to Position 3b for the right hand.

5. **Position 4 - Heart Chakra:** Place your hands on the front and back of the heart. If the person is seated, your hand on the front of the heart should be gently placed under his or her hands. If the person is on a massage table, gently slide one of your hands under the back. Draw SSR energy from the Source of ALL LOVE and send it through your hands into the heart. As this is taking place:

- Intend the flow of energies and appropriate symbols.
- Silently use appropriate empowerment language (three times for each line).
- Silently use the long or short version of the appropriate string of beads.

6. **Position 5 - Third Eye:** Hold your hands on the front and back of the third eye, being sure to include the eyebrows. Draw SSR energy from the Source of ALL LOVE and send it through your hands into the third eye. As this is taking place:

- Intend the flow of energies and appropriate symbols.
- Silently use appropriate empowerment language (three times for each line).
- Silently use the long or short version of the appropriate string of beads.
- *Blow slowly into the crown chakra three times.*

7. **Position 6 - Feet:** If seated, place your hands on the top of the recipient's feet. If on a massage table,

place your hands so that your fingers and/or palms are touching the soles. Draw SSR energy from the Source of ALL LOVE and send it through your hands into the feet. As this is taking place:

- Intend the flow of energies and appropriate symbols.
- Silently use appropriate empowerment language (three times for each line). *(If the person has already received Reiki I, II and/or III, also empower those Reiki degrees in this position as well, since many Reiki lineages do not specifically include the feet. Select the appropriate language from the following: "Reiki I empowerment" three times, "Reiki II empowerment" three times and/or "Reiki III empowerment" three times.)*
- Silently use the long or short version of the appropriate string of beads.

Phase 3

1. **Angelic Light Weaving:** Allow the SSR energy to move through your heart chakra and into your arms and hands. Call on the angelic realms to move your arms and hands above the recipient's physical body and through the subtle bodies in a flowing pattern as guided. Also include the Heart of the Christos symbol and the ankh in your light weaving. Continue for as long as feels appropriate.

2. **Stand behind the person (if on a massage table, stand at the head of the table).** Bring your hands down to the floor and hit the floor with a thump. Then stand back up and raise your hands above your head and clap once loudly. Repeat the thump/clap procedure four times. With each thump and clap, you are reinforcing the anchoring of the person's central column in the center of the Earth and in the heart of the Source of ALL LOVE. The four repetitions cover the physical, emotional, mental and spiritual levels.

3. **Starting from where you have been standing, move 10 times counterclockwise around the**

person. Count on your fingers if necessary to keep your place. Hold your arms out to your sides with the palms facing the person. As you circle, with your right hand gently sprinkle SSR energy into the person's energy field. At the same time, consciously intend with your circling to reinforce and enhance the boundary around the person symbolized by the cosmic egg found in the SKHM Shenu.

4. **Giving Thanks:** Stand in front of the person (or at his or her feet if the recipient is on a massage table) and place your hands together in prayer. Give thanks aloud to the Holy Father God and Mother Goddess and to the angels, guides, teachers, ascended masters and the Source of ALL LOVE for being present during the attunement.

5. **Closing Invocation: If the recipient is sitting, tel**l the person to place the hands on his or her lap. Read aloud the Invocation to the Unified Chakra found in Appendix I, or any other prayer that you feel is appropriate. When the prayer is finished, say aloud to the person:

> *I salute the divine in you. Amen. And so it is.*

6. **Optional:** If you desire, you may now tone with your voice, chime a set of Tibetan bells or play a crystal bowl to complete the ceremony. Sound is very effective in opening any areas of the physical and subtle bodies that still may not be fully flowing. It also helps integrate and balance all levels.

7. **Tell the recipient that your part in the attunement is now complete.** Ask him or her to stay seated or lying on the massage table for a short time to allow the angels, guides, ascended masters and the Source of ALL LOVE to complete the process. Suggest that the person open his or her eyes and get up only when he or she has received an inner prompting that it is time to do so. This may take anywhere from a few minutes to ten or more minutes, depending on the person. Tell the person you are leaving the room and will return in a few minutes.

Appendix XI: Sekhem-Seichim-Reiki Attunement Ceremony "B"

Note to Master Teacher: Attunement Ceremony "B" is identical to Ceremony "A" except for the four modifications discussed in the section entitled Attunement Ceremony "B." Therefore, the discussion of the basic foundation of Ceremony "A" found in the sections entitled Attunement Ceremony "A" as Taught at Facet III and Attunement Ceremony "A" as Supplemented at Facet VII still applies except for these differences.

If you are attuning more than one person at a time, the first six steps of Phase 1 are completed for everyone together as a group. Walk around everyone in one large counterclockwise circle for Step 6. Next complete Step 7 of Phase 1 for the first person and then immediately complete Step 1 of Phase 2 at that person's crown chakra. Then complete these same two steps at the crown chakra for each person before moving to the next person.

When everyone's crown chakra is done, then move from one person to the next completing each person's shoulders. Then do each person's hands, heart and so on until you finish the last position at the feet. In Phase 3, perform the angelic light weaving for each person one at a time. Make the four thumps on the floor and the four claps above your head individually. Then complete the balance of Phase 3 with everyone together as a group.

కు

Phase 1

1. **Have the recipient sit in an upright chair with his or her hands placed palms up on the lap, or lie down on a massage table with arms placed comfortably at the sides.** Be sure the person has taken off his or her watch, glasses and shoes. If desired, play soft music in the background.

If the person is seated, explain that at a certain point in the attunement, you will be moving and gently slapping his or her hands in a particular sequence ending with the hands being placed on the heart (see Positions 3a and 3b). Briefly demonstrate how you will be doing this. Ask the person to keep the hands in this position for the balance of the attunement, if possible. If not, ask the person to gently place the hands back on the lap with palms up.

Explain that the ceremony is a time of silence, receiving and initiation. Suggest that he or she let go of all preconceptions and ideas of what is about to take place and relax, allowing the experience to unfold in the moment. Ask the recipient to close his or her eyes and keep them closed until completion of the ceremony.

2. **Open the central light column.** Ask the person to breathe more deeply and slowly than normal, breathing in up from the lungs, through the shoulders and to the top of the head, then breathing out all the way down to the bottom of the feet. Suggest that the individual do this several times, making the inhaling and exhaling equal in length and creating a circular flow of energy around the entire body.

After the person has begun to relax and quiet down, if the person is seated suggest that he or she become aware of the central light column that connects the chakras and runs parallel to the spine through the middle of the body, from the top of the head to the base of the spine. (If the person is on a massage table, his or her awareness should be brought to the column running vertically from the top of the head to the bottom of the feet.) Ask the person to open and expand the column by gently breathing in and out several times.

Next ask the recipient to visualize his or her feet standing firmly on the Earth while sending the light column down like roots from a tree all the way into the heart of the planet, anchoring it there. Then ask the person to also extend the column above the head all the way through the celestial realms up to the heart of the Source of ALL LOVE, anchoring it there.

As the person maintains the same breathing rhythm, ask him or her to simultaneously breathe the grounding and supportive Earth energies into the column from below and the celestial Heaven energies into the column from above, allowing Heaven and Earth to come together within the heart region. Here the energies blend, merge, balance and unify as One, filling the heart to capacity.

Encourage the person to allow the unified energies to spill over into the entire circulatory system of the physical body, nourishing all the tissues, organs, muscles, bones and cells. Then have the person expand the flow from the heart like a sunburst into the etheric, emotional, mental and spiritual bodies that surround and interpenetrate the physical body.

Once the initial flow through the central light column has been established, the person does not have to concentrate on the breathing and should be encouraged to allow his or her thoughts, feelings and sensations to move wherever the process takes him or her.

3. **Soul mantra:** Stand in front of the person (if seated) or at the head of the table (if on a massage table) and with your arms raised in the air, recite the soul mantra aloud three times. Go through the entire verse before beginning again:

> We are the Soul.
> We are the Monad.
> We are the Light Divine.
> We are Love.
> We are Will.
> We are Perfect Design.

4. **Standing in the same position and speaking aloud, invoke the presence and participation of the angels, guides and teachers of the initiate and yourself as well as the ascended masters and the Source of ALL LOVE.** Invoke them generally or call in certain ones specifically as intuitively guided. Suggest that the initiate silently call in any others he or she wishes to be present.

5. **Standing in the same position, aloud or silently say:**

> *Thank you. Thank you. Thank you, Holy Father God and Mother Goddess for the privilege of giving this empowerment.*

6. **Starting from where you have been standing, move eight times counterclockwise around the recipient.** Count on your fingers if necessary to keep your place. Hold your palms in the air, facing them toward the recipient as you walk. Say silently:

> *You, [initiate's name], are free to accept or reject this Sekhem-Seichim-Reiki empowerment. Sekhem-Seichim-Reiki is a harmonizing, healing, balancing and loving universal energy of the Christ Consciousness and the I AM Presence. I ask the healing god Thoth and the goddess Isis to make every moment of this attunement equal to millions of years of healing, wholing and loving.*

7. **Statement of intent and invitation:** Stand in back of the recipient with your hands on top of his or her head, fingers together. Silently say a statement of intent and make an invitation to the Source of ALL LOVE as follows:

> *This is an attunement for SSR Facet(s) (state those to be included), together with the SSR symbol(s) (state those to be included). With great appreciation and love, we also welcome and invite in whatever additional energy and light transmissions this person is ready to receive directly from the Source of ALL LOVE.*

Phase 2

1. **Position 1 - Top of Head:** With your hands still on top of the recipient's head, draw SSR energy from the Source of ALL LOVE and send it through your hands into the head. As this is taking place:

- Intend the flow of energies and appropriate symbols.
- Silently say "ALL LOVE empowerment" (at least three times).
- Silently use the long or short version of the appropriate string of beads.

2. **Position 2 - Shoulders:** Stand in back of the person with your hands on his or her shoulders, fingers together. Draw SSR energy from the Source of ALL LOVE and send it through your hands into the shoulders. As this is taking place:

- Intend the flow of energies and appropriate symbols.
- Silently say "ALL LOVE empowerment" (at least three times).
- Silently use the long or short version of the appropriate string of beads.

3. **Position 3a - Fingertips (if seated):** Stand in front of the person and silently guide the recipient to hold his or her hands in front of the heart in prayer position, with the fingers and thumbs together. Place one of your hands around his or her wrists. Cup your other hand over the person's fingertips and thumbs. Draw SSR energy from the Source of ALL LOVE and send it through your hands into the recipient's fingertips and thumbs. As this is taking place:

- Intend the flow of energies and appropriate symbols.
- Silently say "ALL LOVE empowerment" (at least three times).
- *For this position only, you do not need to use the string of beads, as this is completed for the entire hand area with Position 3b.*

Position 3a - Fingertips (if on a massage table): Stand to the left side of the person and place one of your hands around his or her wrist. Cup your other hand over the person's fingertips and thumb. Draw SSR energy from the Source of ALL LOVE and send it through your hands into the recipient's fingertips and thumb. As this is taking place:

- Intend the flow of energies and appropriate symbols.
- Silently say "ALL LOVE empowerment" (at least three times).
- *For this position only, you do not have to use the string of beads, as this is completed for the entire hand area with Position 3b.*

Now complete Position 3b below for the left hand and then move to the right side of the person and complete Position 3a for the right hand per the above. Then go on to Position 3b for the right hand.

4. **Position 3b - Palms and Back of Hands (if seated):** While still standing in front of the recipient, move his or hands so that they are held comfortably side by side, cupped with the palms open and at waist height. Hold the palm of your non-dominant hand under the person's two open and cupped hands so that your palm is placed behind and up against the back of the person's hands. Draw SSR energy from the Source of ALL LOVE and send it through your hand into the back of the recipient's hands. Simultaneously, send SSR energy from the Source of ALL LOVE through your third eye into the person's palms. As this is taking place:

- Intend the flow of energies and appropriate symbols.
- Silently say "ALL LOVE empowerment" (at least three times).
- Silently use the long or short version of the appropriate string of beads.
- *Blow on the cupped palms three times.*

Gently place one of the person's palms over the heart chakra. Take the other open palm and place your non-dominant hand underneath it to support the next motion. Using your dominant hand, flatten out the person's open palm. Then gently but firmly slap the open hand, holding your slapping hand flat on his or her palm for a few seconds before beginning again. Slap the palm a total of three times. Then reverse the person's hands and follow the same procedure. When you are finished with the person's second hand, place it across the other one, over the heart.

Position 3b - Palms and Back of Hands (if on a massage table): While still standing to the left side of the recipient, gently move his or her left hand so that it is open with the palm up. Hold the palm of your non-dominant hand under the person's open hand so that your palm is placed behind and up against the back of the person's hand. Draw SSR energy from the Source of ALL LOVE and send it through your hand into the back of the recipient's hand. Simultaneously, send SSR energy from the Source of ALL LOVE through your third eye into the person's left palm. As this is taking place:

- Intend the flow of energies and appropriate symbols.
- Silently say "ALL LOVE empowerment" (at least three times).
- Silently use the long or short version of the appropriate string of beads.
- *Blow on the cupped palm three times.*

After completing Position 3b for the left hand, move to the right side of the person and complete Position 3a for the right hand. Then come back to Position 3b for the right hand.

5. **Position 4 - Heart Chakra:** Place your hands on the front and back of the heart. If the person is seated, your hand on the front of the heart should be gently placed under his or her hands. If the person is on a massage table, gently slide one of your hands under the back. Draw SSR energy from the Source of ALL LOVE and send it through your hands into the heart. As this is taking place:

- Intend the flow of energies and appropriate symbols.
- Silently say "ALL LOVE empowerment" (at least three times).
- Silently use the long or short version of the appropriate string of beads.

6. **Position 5 - Third Eye:** Hold your hands on the front and back of the third eye, being sure to include the eyebrows. Draw SSR energy from the Source of ALL LOVE and send it through your hands into the third eye. As this is taking place:

- Intend the flow of energies and appropriate symbols.
- Silently say "ALL LOVE empowerment" (at least three times).
- Silently use the long or short version of the appropriate string of beads.
- *Blow slowly into the crown chakra three times.*

7. **Position 6 - Feet:** If seated, place your hands on the top of the recipient's feet. If on a massage table, place your hands so that your fingers and/or palms are touching the soles. Draw SSR energy from the Source of ALL LOVE and send it through your hands into the feet. As this is taking place:

- Intend the flow of energies and appropriate symbols.
- Silently say "ALL LOVE empowerment" (at least three times).
- Silently use the long or short version of the appropriate string of beads.

Phase 3

1. **Angelic Light Weaving:** Allow the SSR energy to move through your heart chakra and into your arms and hands. Call on the angelic realms to move your arms and hands above the recipient's physical body and through the subtle bodies in a flowing pattern as guided. Also include the Heart of the Christos

symbol and the ankh in your light weaving. Continue for as long as feels appropriate.

2. **Stand behind the person (if on a massage table, stand at the head of the table).** Bring your hands down to the floor and hit the floor with a thump. Then stand back up and raise your hands above your head and clap once loudly. Repeat the thump/clap procedure four times. With each thump and clap, you are reinforcing the anchoring of the person's central column in the center of the Earth and in the heart of the Source of ALL LOVE. The four repetitions cover the physical, emotional, mental and spiritual levels.

3. **Starting from where you have been standing, move 10 times counterclockwise around the person.** Count on your fingers if necessary to keep your place. Hold your arms out to your sides with the palms facing the person. As you circle, with your right hand gently sprinkle SSR energy into the person's energy field. At the same time, consciously intend with your circling to reinforce and enhance the boundary around the person symbolized by the cosmic egg found in the SKHM Shenu.

4. **Giving Thanks:** Stand in front of the person (or at his or her feet if the recipient is on a massage table) and place your hands together in prayer. Give thanks aloud to the Holy Father God and Mother Goddess and to the angels, guides, teachers, ascended masters and the Source of ALL LOVE for being present during the attunement.

5. **Closing Invocation:** If the recipient is sitting, tell the person to place the hands on his or her lap. Read aloud the Invocation to the Unified Chakra found in Appendix I, or any other prayer that you feel is appropriate. When the prayer is finished, say aloud to the person:

I salute the divine in you. Amen. And so it is.

6. **Optional:** If you desire, you may now tone with your voice, chime a set of Tibetan bells or play a crystal bowl to complete the ceremony. Sound is very effective in opening any areas of the physical and subtle bodies that still may not be fully flowing. It also helps integrate and balance all levels.

7. **Tell the recipient that your part in the attunement is now complete.** Ask him or her to stay seated or lying on the massage table for a short time to allow the angels, guides, ascended masters and the Source of ALL LOVE to complete the process. Suggest that the person open his or her eyes and get up only when he or she has received an inner prompting that it is time to do so. This may take anywhere from a few minutes to ten or more minutes, depending on the person. Tell the person you are leaving the room and will return in a few minutes.

Bibliography

Ascension and Light Body

Bailey, Alice A. *The Consciousness of the Atom*. New York: Lucis Publishing Company, 1993.

——————. *The Destiny of the Nations*. New York: Lucis Publishing Company, 1978.

——————. *Discipleship in the New Age*. Vol. 1. New York: Lucis Publishing Company, 1979.

——————. *Discipleship in the New Age*. Vol. 2. New York: Lucis Publishing Company, 1979.

——————. *Education in the New Age*. Lucis Publishing Company, 1974.

——————. *The Externalisation of the Hierarchy*. New York: Lucis Publishing Company, 1989.

——————. *From Bethlehem to Calvary: The Initiations of Jesus*. New York: Lucis Publishing Company, 1976.

——————. *From Intellect to Intuition*. New York: Lucis Publishing Company, 1987.

——————. *Glamour: A World Problem*. New York: Lucis Publishing Company, 1978.

——————. *Initiation, Human and Solar*. New York: Lucis Publishing Company, 1992.

——————. *Letters on Occult Meditation*. New York: Lucis Publishing Company, 1979.

——————. *The Light of the Soul: Its Science and Effect: A Paraphrase of the Yoga Sutras of Patañjali*. New York: Lucis Publishing Company, 1988.

——————. *Problems of Humanity*. New York: Lucis Publishing Company, 1993.

——————. *The Reappearance of the Christ*. New York: Lucis Publishing Company,1979.

——————. *The Soul and Its Mechanism: The Problem of Psychology*. New York: Lucis Publishing Company, 1987.

——————. *Telepathy and the Etheric Vehicle*. New York: Lucis Publishing Company, 1986.

——————. *A Treatise on Cosmic Fire*. New York: Lucis Publishing Company, 1995.

——————. *A Treatise on the Seven Rays: Volume 1, Esoteric Psychology*. New York: Lucis Publishing Company, 1962.

——————. *A Treatise on the Seven Rays: Volume 2, Esoteric Psychology*. New York: Lucis Publishing Company, 1975.

——————. *A Treatise on the Seven Rays: Volume 3, Esoteric Astrology*. New York: Lucis Publishing Company, 1974.

——————. *A Treatise on the Seven Rays: Volume 4, Esoteric Healing*. New York: Lucis Publishing Company, 1953.

——————. *A Treatise on the Seven Rays: Volume 5, The Rays and the Initiations*. New York: Lucis Publishing Company, 1962.

——————. *A Treatise on White Magic: or The Way of the Disciple*. New York: Lucis Publishing Company, 1991.

——————. *The Unfinished Autobiography of Alice A. Bailey*. New York: Lucis Publishing Company, 1987.

Cooper, Diana. *A Little Light on Ascension*. Forres, Scotland: Findhorn Press, 1997.

Everett, Julianne. *Heart Initiation: Preparing for Conscious Ascension*. Livermore, Calif.: Oughten House Publications, 1996.

Feurst, Irving and Virginia Essene. *Energy Blessings From the Stars: Seven Initiations*. Santa Clara, Calif.: S.E.E. Publishing Company, 1998.

Ford-Crenshaw, Ruth. *Design Your Intention: An Experience of Embodying Source*. Livermore, Calif.: Inner Eye Books, 1997.

Grattan, Brian. *Mahatma I & II: The I Am Presence*. Sedona, Ariz.: Light Technology Publishing, 1994.

Kenyon, Tom and Virginia Essene. Santa Clara, Calif.: *The Hathor Material: Messages from an Ascended Civilization*. S.E.E. Publishing Company, 1996.

Mann, John and Lar Short. *The Body of Light: History and Practical Techniques for Awakening Your Subtle Body*. New York: Globe Press Books, 1990.

McClure, Janet, channeling Vywamus and Others. *Prelude to Ascension: Tools for Transformation*. Sedona, Ariz.: Light Technology Publishing, 1996.

Stevenson, Sandy. *The Awakener: The Time Is Now*. Bath, United Kingdom: Gateway Books, 1997.

Stone, Joshua David. *The Ascended Masters Light the Way: Beacons of Ascension*. Sedona, Ariz.: Light Technology Publishing, 1995.

—————. *A Beginner's Guide to The Path of Ascension*. Sedona, Ariz.: Light Technology Publishing, 1998.

—————. *Beyond Ascension: How to Complete the Seven Levels of Initiation*. Sedona, Ariz.: Light Technology Publishing, 1995.

—————. *The Complete Ascension Manual: How to Achieve Ascension in this Lifetime*. Sedona, Ariz.: Light Technology Publishing, 1994.

—————. *Cosmic Ascension: Your Cosmic Map Home*. Sedona, Ariz.: Light Technology Publishing, 1997.

—————. *Golden Keys to Ascension and Healing: Revelations of Sai Baba and the Ascended Masters*. Sedona, Ariz.: Light Technology Publishing, 1998.

—————. *Hidden Mysteries: ETs, Ancient Mystery Schools and Ascension*. Sedona, Ariz.: Light Technology Publishing, 1995.

—————. *How to Teach Ascension Classes*. Sedona, Ariz.: Light Technology Publishing, 1998.

—————. *Manual for Planetary Leadership*. Sedona, Ariz.: Light Technology Publishing, 1998.

—————. *Revelations of a Melchizedek Initiate*. Sedona, Ariz.: Light Technology Publishing, 1998.

—————. *Soul Psychology: Keys to Ascension*. Sedona, Ariz.: Light Technology Publishing, 1994.

—————. *Your Ascension Mission: Embracing Your Puzzle Piece*. Sedona, Ariz.: Light Technology Publishing, 1998.

Stubbs, Tony. *An Ascension Handbook: Material Channeled From Serapis*. Lithia Springs, Ga.: New Leaf, 1999.

Tashira Tachi-ren, channeling Archangel Ariel. *What Is Lightbody?* Livermore, Calif.: Oughten House Publications, 1995.

Two Disciples. *The Rainbow Bridge: First and Second Phases, Link with the Soul, Purification*. Danville, Calif.: Triune Foundation, 1994.

Divine Guidance

Bunick, Nick. *In God's Truth*. Charlottesville, Va.: Hampton Roads Publishing Company, Inc., 1998.

Ingram, Julia and G.W. Hardin. *The Messengers, A True Story of Angelic Presence and the Return to the Age of Miracles*. New York: Pocket Books, 1997.

Milanovich, Norma, and Shirley McCune. *The Light Shall Set You Free*. Albuquerque, N.Mex.: Athena Publishing, 1996.

Walsch, Neale Donald. *Conversations with God: An Uncommon Dialogue*. Charlottesville, Va.: Hampton Roads Publishing Company, Inc., 1995.

—————. *Conversations with God : An Uncommon Dialogue Book 2*. Charlottesville, Va.: Hampton Roads Publishing Company, Inc., 1997.

—————. *Conversations with God : An Uncommon Dialogue Book 3*. Charlottesville, Va.: Hampton Roads Publishing Company, Inc., 1998.

Virtue, Doreen. *Angel Therapy: Healing Messages for Every Area of Your Life*. Carlsbad, Calif.: Hay House, Inc., 1997.

—————. *Divine Guidance: How to Have a Dialogue With God and Your Guardian Angels*. Los Angeles: Renaissance Books, 1998.

—————. *The Lightworker's Way: Awakening Your Spiritual Power to Know and Heal*. Carlsbad, Calif.: Hay House, Inc., 1997.

General Interest

Ashby, Muata. *The Serpent Power: The Ancient Egyptian Mystical Wisdom of the Inner Life Force*. Miami: Cruzian Mystic Books, 1997.

Ashby, Muata and Karen Clarke-Ashby. *Egyptian Yoga: The Philosophy of Enlightenment.* Miami: Cruzian Mystic Books, 1995.

—————. *Egyptian Yoga, Vol. 2: The Supreme Wisdom of Enlightenment.* Miami: Cruzian Mystic Books, 1998.

Bach, Richard. *Jonathan Livingston Seagull: A Story.* New York: Avon Books, 1973.

Berges, John. *Sacred Vessel of The Mysteries: The Great Invocation - Word of Power, Gift of Love.* Northfield, N.J.: Planetwork Press, 1997.

Braden, Gregg. *Awakening to Zero Point: The Collective Initiation.* Bellevue, Wash.: Radio Bookstore Press, 1997.

—————. *Walking Between the Worlds: The Science of Compassion.* Bellevue, Wash.: Radio Bookstore Press, 1997.

Bunson, Margaret. *A Dictionary of Ancient Egypt.* New York: Oxford University Press, 1995.

Cooper, J.C. *An Illustrated Encyclopaedia of Traditional Symbols.* London: Thames and Hudson, Ltd., 1978.

—————. *Symbolism: The Universal Language.* Wellingborough, England: The Aquarian Press, 1982.

Cox, Robert. *The Pillar of Celestial Fire: The Lost Science of The Ancient Seers Rediscovered.* Fairfield, Iowa: Sunstar Publishing, Ltd., 1997.

Dass, Ram, and Mirabai Bush. *Compassion in Action: Setting Out on The Path of Service.* New York: Bell Tower, 1992.

Fideler, David. *Jesus Christ, Sun of God: Ancient Cosmology and Early Christian Symbolism.* Wheaton, Ill: Theosophical Publishing House, 1993.

Foundation for Inner Peace. *A Course in Miracles.* Mill Valley, Calif.: Foundation for Inner Peace, 1992.

Hall, Manly P. *The Secret Teachings of All Ages: An Encyclopedic Outline of Masonic, Hermetic, Qabbalistic and Rosicrucian Symbolical Philosophy: Being an Interpretation of the Secret Teachings Concealed Within the Rituals, Allegories and Mysteries of All Ages.* Los Angeles: The Philosophical Research Society, Inc., 1988.

Linn, Denise. *Sacred Space: Clearing and Enhancing the Energy of Your Home.* New York: Ballantine Books, 1996.

Masters, Robert. *The Goddess Sekhmet: Psychospiritual Exercises of the Fifth Way.* St. Paul, Minn.: Llewellyn Publications, 1991.

Melchizedek, Drunvalo. *The Ancient Secret of The Flower of Life: An Edited Transcript of The Flower of Life Workshop Presented Live to Mother Earth from 1985 to 1994, Vol. 1.* Sedona, Ariz.: Light Technology Publishing, 1998.

Metford, J.C.J. *Dictionary of Christian Lore and Legend.* New York: Thames and Hudson, Inc., 1983.

Page, Ken. *The Way It Works.* Bastrop, Tx.: Clear Light Arts, 1999.

Roberts, Alison. *Hathor Rising: The Power of the Goddess in Ancient Egypt.* Rochester, Vt.: Inner Traditions International, 1997.

Schwaller de Lubicz, Isha and Lucie Lamy. *Her-Bak: Egyptian Initiate.* Rochester, Vt.: Inner Traditions International, 1978.

Shaw, Ian and Paul Nicholson. *British Museum Dictionary of Ancient Egypt.* London: British Museum Press, 1995.

Tresidder, Jack. *Dictionary of Symbols: An Illustrated Guide to Traditional Images, Icons and Emblems.* San Francisco: Chronicle Books, 1998.

Trout, Susan S. *Born to Serve: The Evolution of the Soul through Service.* Alexandria, Va.: Three Roses Press, 1997.

Wilkinson, Richard H. *Symbol & Magic in Egyptian Art.* London: Thames and Hudson, Ltd., 1994.

Williamson, Marianne. *A Return to Love: Reflections on the Principles of A Course In Miracles.* New York: HarperPerennial, 1996.

Wing, R.L. *The I Ching Workbook.* New York: Doubleday, 1979.

Healing and The Human Energy System

Brennan, Barbara Ann. *Hands of Light: A Guide to Healing through the Human Energy Field: A New Paradigm for the Human Being in Health, Relationship, and Disease.* New York: Bantam Books, 1988.

——————. *Light Emerging: The Journey of Personal Healing.* New York: Bantam Books, 1993.

Bruyere, Rosalyn L. and Jeanne Farrens. *Wheels of Light: Chakras, Auras, and the Healing Energy of the Body.* New York: Simon & Schuster, 1994.

Carlson, Richard and Benjamin Shield, eds. *Healers on Healing.* Los Angeles: Jeremy P. Tarcher, Inc., 1989.

Gawain, Shakti. *The Path of Transformation: How Healing Ourselves Can Change the World.* Mill Valley, Calif.: Nataraj Publishing, 1993.

Goldner, Diane. *Infinite Grace: Where the Worlds of Science and Spiritual Healing Meet.* Charlottesville, Va.: Hampton Roads Publishing Company, Inc., 1999.

Greenwell, Bonnie. *Energies of Transformation: A Guide to the Kundalini Process.* Cupertino, Calif.: Shakti River Press, 1990.

Hay, Louise L. *Heal Your Body: The Mental Causes for Physical Illness and the Metaphysical Way to Overcome Them.* Santa Monica, Calif.: Hay House, Inc., 1984.

——————. *You Can Heal Your Life.* Santa Monica, Calif.: Hay House, Inc., 1984.

Hay, Louise L., and Glenn Kolb. *Love Yourself, Heal Your Life Workbook.* Santa Monica, Calif.: Hay House, Inc., 1990.

Hay, Louise L., and Linda Tomchin. *The Power is Within You.* Carson, Calif.: Hay House, Inc., 1991.

Johnson, Robert A. *Owning Your Own Shadow: Understanding the Dark Side of the Psyche.* San Francisco: HarperSanFrancisco, 1991.

Leadbeater, C.W. *Man Visible and Invisible; Examples of Different Types of Men as Seen by Means of Trained Clairvoyance.* Wheaton, Ill.: The Theosophical Publishing House, 1925.

Motoyama, Hiroshi. *Theories of the Chakras: Bridge to Higher Consciousness.* Wheaton, Ill.: The Theosophical Publishing House, 1981.

Myss, Caroline. *Anatomy of The Spirit: The Seven Stages of Power and Healing.* New York: Harmony Books, 1996.

——————. *Why People Don't Heal and How They Can.* New York: Harmony Books, 1997.

Page, Ken and Shirley Ann Holly. *Multidimensional Cellular Healing: Philosophy and Applications, Volume 1.* Bastrop, Tx.: Clear Light Arts, 1996.

——————. *Multidimensional Cellular Healing: Mastery Guide, Volume 2.* Bastrop, Tx.: Clear Light Arts, 1996.

Paulson, Genevieve Lewis. *Kundalini and The Chakras: A Practical Manual - Evolution in This Lifetime.* St. Paul, Minn.: Llewellyn Publications, 1991.

Pearsall, Paul. *The Heart's Code: Tapping the Wisdom and Power of Our Heart Energy.* New York: Broadway Books, 1998.

Schwarz, Jack. *Human Energy Systems.* New York: E.P. Dutton, 1980.

Trout, Susan S. *To See Differently: Personal Growth and Being of Service Through Attitudinal Healing.* Washington, D.C.: Three Roses Press, 1990.

Walsh, Roger, and Frances Vaughan, eds. *Paths Beyond Ego: The Transpersonal Vision.* Los Angeles: Jeremy P. Tarcher, Inc., 1993.

Zweig, Connie, and Jeremiah Abrams, eds. *Meeting the Shadow: The Hidden Power of the Dark Side of Human Nature.* Los Angeles: Jeremy P. Tarcher, Inc., 1991.

Healing With Sound

Beaulieu, John. *Music and Sound in the Healing Arts: An Energy Approach.* Barrytown, N.Y.: Station Hill Press, 1987.

Cousto. *The Cosmic Octave: Origin of Harmony, Planets, Tones, Colors, the Power of Inherent Vibrations.* Mendocino, Calif.: LifeRhythm, 1988.

Crowley, Brian, and Esther Crowley. *Words of Power: Sacred Sounds of East & West*. St. Paul, Minn.: Llewellyn Publications, 1991.

Gardner, Kay. *Music as Medicine: The Art & Science of Healing With Sound*. Boulder, Colo.: Sounds True, 1998. Six cassette tapes plus study guide.

—————. *Sounding the Inner Landscape: Music as Medicine*. Rockport, Mass.: Element Books Ltd., 1997.

Goldman, Jonathan. *Healing Sounds: The Power of Harmonics*. Rockport, Mass.: Element Books Ltd., 1996.

—————. *Shifting Frequencies*. Sedona, Ariz.: Light Technology Publishing, 1998.

Keyes, Laurel Elizabeth. *Toning, The Creative Power of the Voice*. Marina del Rey, Calif.: DeVorss & Company, 1973.

Rachele, Rollin. *Overtone Singing Study Guide*. 2nd ed. Amsterdam, The Netherlands: Cryptic Voices Productions, 1996. Includes CD with exercises.

Legal and Business

Meengs, Karen L. *The Goddess As Entrepreneur: Right-Brained Tools for Left-Brained Businesses*. Great Falls, Va.: Over The Cliff Publications, Inc., 1998. Cassette tape set with materials.

Rebirthing and Conscious Breathwork

Frissell, Bob. *Nothing In This Book Is True, But It's Exactly How Things Are: The Esoteric Meaning of the Monuments on Mars*. Berkeley, Calif.: Frog Ltd., 1994.

—————. *Something in This Book is True ...* Berkeley, Calif.: Frog, Ltd., 1997.

Grof, Stanislav, and Hal Zina Bennett. *The Holotropic Mind: Three Levels of Human Consciousness and How They Shape Our Lives*. San Francisco: HarperSanFrancisco, 1992.

Hendricks, Gay. *Conscious Breathing: Breathwork for Health, Stress Release and Personal Mastery*. New York: Bantam Books, 1995.

Leonard, Jim, and Phil Laut. *Vivation: The Science of Enjoying All of Your Life*. Cincinnati: Vivation Publications, 1991.

Minett, Gunnel. *Breath & Spirit: Rebirthing as a Healing Technique*. London: Aquarian/Thorsons, 1994.

Orr, Leonard. *Breaking the Death Habit: The Science of Everlasting Life*. Berkeley, Calif.: Frog Ltd., 1998.

Orr, Leonard, and Sondra Ray. *Rebirthing in the New Age*. Berkeley, Calif.: Celestial Arts, 1983.

Ray, Sondra. *Celebration of Breath (Rebirthing, Book II): How to Survive Anything and Heal Your Body*. Berkeley, Calif.: Celestial Arts, 1986.

—————. *Loving Relationships: The Secrets of a Great Relationship*. Berkeley, Calif.: Celestial Arts, 1980.

Sisson, Colin P. *Rebirthing Made Easy: A Gateway to Self Knowledge, Aliveness and Compassion*. Santa Monica, Calif.: Hay House, Inc., 1987.

Reiki and Seichim/SKHM

Arnold, Larry E., and Sandra K. Nevius. *The Reiki Handbook: A Manual for Students and Therapists of the Usui Shiko Ryoho System of Healing*. Harrisburg, Pa.: PSI Press, 1982.

Burack, Marsha. *Reiki, Healing Yourself and Others: A Photo-Instructional Art Book*. Encinitas, Calif.: Lo Ro Productions, Reiki Healing Institute, 1995. Includes a section on Seichim.

Mitchell, Karyn. *Reiki: A Torch in Daylight*. Sedona, Ariz.: Mind Rivers Publications, 1994.

—————. *Reiki: Beyond the Usui System*. Daysville Ore.: Mind Rivers Publications, 1994.

Petter, Frank Arjava. *Reiki: The Legacy of Dr. Usui: Rediscovered Documents on the Origins and Developments of the Reiki System, as Well as New Aspects of the Reiki Energy*. Twin Lakes, Wis.: Lotus Light Publications, 1998.

—————. *Reiki Fire: New Information about the Origins of the Reiki Power, A Complete Manual*. Twin Lakes, Wis.: Lotus Light Publications, 1998.

Rowland, Amy Z. *Traditional Reiki for Our Times: Practical Methods for Personal and Planetary Healing*. Rochester, Vt: Healing Arts Press, 1998. Includes a section on Seichim.

Shewmaker, Diane Ruth. *ALL LOVE FOR TEACHERS: A Manual for Teaching Sekhem-Seichim-Reiki and SKHM*. Beaverton, Ore.: Celestial Wellspring Publications, 2000. Forthcoming.

Stein, Diane. *Essential Reiki: A Complete Guide to An Ancient Healing Art*. Freedom, Calif.: The Crossing Press, Inc., 1996.

Index

Contact Information

Classes, Workshops, Speaking Engagements and Healing Sessions with Diane Ruth Shewmaker

SSR and SKHM classes led by me are scheduled throughout the United States. Workshops and speaking engagements on other spiritual growth and metaphysical topics of interest are also periodically scheduled on topics such as ascension; light body and sacred geometry activation; awakening the unified heart; working with angels and the ascended masters; and rebirthing. Announcements of these classes and workshops can be found on my website at www.celestialwellspring.com. As well, healing sessions are available, both in person and at a distance.

If you wish to be included on my mailing list, please send your name, address, telephone number and e-mail address to:

Diane Ruth Shewmaker	Phone:	800-966-5857 • 503-469-9292
Celestial Wellspring Publications	Fax:	503-469-9393
6107 SW Murray Blvd., PMB213	E-mail:	awakener@celestialwellspring.com
Beaverton, Oregon 97008-4467	Web:	www.celestialwellspring.com

Additional information about SKHM classes and becoming a certified teacher of SKHM may be found at www.SKHM.com. The site also includes a current list of certified SKHM teachers.

Contacting Patrick Zeigler, Tom Seaman & Marsha Nityankari Burack

Patrick Zeigler
853 Hutcheson Lane
Blacksburg, Virginia 24060
540-552-8267
Seichim@aol.com

Tom Seaman
t-om@efn.org

Marsha Nityankari Burack
The Reiki Healing Institute
449 Santa Fe Drive, #303
Encinitas, California 92024
760-436-1865

Contacting the Artists

Lesley Stoune
Chameleon Soul
9406 Canton Avenue
Lubbock, Texas 79423
806-745-8738
806-748-7877 (fax)
artisan@chameleonsoul.com
www.chameleonsoul.com

Wendy Bush Hackney
Spirit Journey Enterprises
109 Discovery Lane
Lexington, Virginia 24450
540-463-7030
540-463-7693 (fax)

About the Author

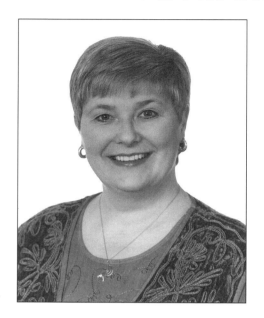

Diane Ruth Shewmaker

Diane Ruth Shewmaker is the creator of the Sekhem-Seichim-Reiki healing matrix which is the subject of this Guidebook. Already a Seichim and Reiki Master, Diane channeled new information in 1997 about the third component of the matrix, which she was guided to call Sekhem, as well as information on how the three energies work together as a unified, full-spectrum healing system. This led her to combine these three infinite expressions of universal love as Sekhem-Seichim-Reiki (SSR).

Diane has been an avid student and teacher of traditional, holistic and metaphysical healing arts for more than 20 years. She is a licensed psychotherapist who brings a rich background and the experience of her personal soul path to her work as a highly gifted and skilled spiritual and intuitive counselor, healer, teacher, channel, author and universal lightworker. This background includes general, transpersonal and Jungian psychology; psychosynthesis; Gestalt theory and practice; hypnotherapy; meditation; *A Course in Miracles*; various body-centered modalities; and other complementary methods of healing such as rebirthing, attitudinal healing and energy work.

Over the years, Diane's professional and volunteer counseling experience has embraced working with individuals, couples and groups having concerns about balancing body, mind and spirit; life transitions and changes, grief and loss; chronic and terminal illness; relationship issues; childhood abuse; codependence and addictions; depression; anxiety; and stress. Diane has also counseled people seeking to find their life's work and purpose; to open greater access to their creative talents and spiritual gifts; and to connect more deeply with their spirit guides, angels, the ascended masters and the Source of ALL LOVE.

In searching for a way to help others deal with such issues (as well as in pursuing her personal healing), Diane took up the study of the human energy system and how its physical, emotional, mental and spiritual components influence and interact with each other to create either a state of health or a state of "dis-ease." In the process, she became a Practitioner and Master Teacher of several energy work systems that specifically address the healing process at all of these levels. These systems include: SSR; Seichim; Isis Seichim; Traditional Usui, Tibetan and Contemporary Reiki; and Karuna Reiki®. Diane is also a certified teacher of SKHM, having completed a one-year training course with Patrick Zeigler, who brought Seichim/SKHM to the world from Egypt.

Further studies have been completed with Ken Page, the developer of Heart and Soul Healing® (also known as Multidimensional Cellular Healing®), to become a Certified Practitioner of this powerful modality. Diane has also received training in the psychic and spiritual healing arts from Doreen Virtue, Ph.D., and is a Certified Spiritual Counselor (see www.angeltherapy.com). As well, Diane is a Certified Instructor and Practitioner of a dynamic self-development and spiritual healing system called Kofutu Touch Healing and Kofutu Absent Formula Healing. She has also studied Hawaiian Kahuna healing.

In addition to teaching classes throughout the United States in those healing modalities already mentioned where she is a Master Teacher or Certified Instructor, Diane leads seminars and workshops nationally and is available for speaking engagements on a variety of metaphysical and spiritual growth topics such as ascension; light body and sacred geometry activation; awakening the unified heart; working with angels and the ascended masters; and rebirthing.

Diane's professional background also includes nearly 25 years of human resource development and administrative experience within nonprofit, legal and public accounting organizations. Within these various settings, Diane worked successfully with management and staff at all levels. She also designed and led trainings and work discussion groups in such topics as stress reduction and life management skills; time management; understanding and coping with organizational change; communication and interpersonal skills; conflict management; team building; diversity training; optimum wellness; and downsizing. Her last position in a corporate setting was as Director of Administration and Human Resources for a nonprofit organization in Washington, D.C.

Diane holds a master of arts degree in education and human development, with a major in community mental health counseling, and a bachelor of business administration degree in human resource management. Both are from The George Washington University in Washington, D.C. She is a licensed psychotherapist in several states and is a professional member of the American Counseling Association and the American Mental Health Counseling Association. She is also an ordained nondenominational minister in the Order of Melchizedek. Diane currently resides with her husband and her cat Ganesha in Beaverton, Oregon.

❧

Sharing Your Sekhem-Seichim-Reiki and SKHM Story

I am always interested in comments, suggestions or any wisdom from you regarding your SSR and SKHM experiences. Please feel free to share this information with me by e-mail or U.S. mail. Please include your name, address, telephone number and e-mail address in your correspondence. Please send the information to:

Diane Ruth Shewmaker
Celestial Wellspring Publications
6107 SW Murray Boulevard, PMB213
Beaverton, Oregon 97008-4467
800-966-5857 • 503-469-9292
503-469-9393 (fax)
awakener@celestialwellspring.com
www.celestialwellspring.com

About the Designer

Lesley Stoune is first and foremost a metaphysician; she is also a fine artist and expresses much of her spiritual understandings through her artwork. She was born with a passionate desire to give expression to the deep emotional and spiritual energies that have always been an intimate part of her life. One of the important ways she does this is visually. First with crayons and later with charcoal, pastels and ultimately a Macintosh computer, Lesley learned the ways in which color, line and form combine to give visual expression to universal energies. Her strong intuitive understanding of this process is something she now relies on everyday as both an energy worker and graphic artist.

Another important tool that Lesley uses in her work is her understanding of how artwork, design and words interact. She believes that in any successfully crafted project the design and illustrations must embrace and accentuate the content allowing it to reach out to the reader unencumbered by flashy layouts or disharmonious colors. This is truly a case where the total energetic and visual effect is greater than the sum of the parts.

She feels that her understanding of this process was clarified and accentuated in college where she had the freedom to write her own degree plan. At Texas Tech University, she combined studies of Fine Art, Design, Journalism, Technical Writing and English Literature into a bachelor's program that brought integration of words and design into focus for her. This program also helped her to hone her writing skills and learn to "paint" with words just as she does with color.

Lesley has worked in the graphic arts field for more than 13 years and currently savors the freedom of working from home. Chameleon Design Studio is just one aspect of her many interests, which she combines under the name Chameleon Soul. She enjoys working on a variety of expressive projects including creative art and writing; designing and illustrating books, logos and other business materials; and designing websites.

Lesley is also dedicated to community building and teaching. She is the sponsor of a monthly lecture/discussion group called the Metaphysical Mixer, and publishes a monthly newsletter for her local metaphysical community. She and her husband C.D. Stoune received the SSR Master Teacher attunement from Diane Ruth Shewmaker in the spring of 1999 and have enjoyed sharing the energy and knowledge with others in weekend classes and healing sessions. Lesley is also a gifted psychic energy reader and Rune master. She considers her energetic healing and spiritual counseling work to be among the most rewarding and enjoyable parts of her life.

Lesley Stoune
Chameleon Soul
9406 Canton Avenue
Lubbock, Texas 79423
806-745-8738
806-748-7877 (fax)
artisan@chameleonsoul.com
www.chameleonsoul.com

Ordering Information

Additional copies of ALL LOVE and prints of The SKHM Shenu may be purchased as follows:

SHENU PRINTS

❏ 8″ x 10″ SKHM Shenu print

The shenu is printed in full color with a description and instructions for its use in meditation printed on the back. This beautiful image is laminated and is also suitable for framing.

$8.00 each ($2.50 S&H in U.S. / $6.00 foreign)

❏ 18″ x 24″ SKHM Shenu poster

This image is printed in full color and mailed in a protective cardboard tube. Suitable for framing.

$20.00 each ($4.00 S&H in U.S. / $10.00 foreign)

BOOKS

❏ ALL LOVE: A Guidebook for Healing With Sekhem-Sechim-Reiki and SKHM

$18.95 each

❏ ALL LOVE FOR TEACHERS: A Manual for Teaching Sekhem-Seichim-Reiki and SKHM

$18.95 each (forthcoming in early 2000)

Shipping & Handling for books:	U.S. Priority Mail:	$6	Airmail to Canada:	$12
(Prices are per book. All others	UPS Ground in U.S.:	$12	Airmail to Europe:	$16
gauge postage by these.)	Overnight Delivery:	please call	Airmail to Australia:	$21

PLEASE CALL ABOUT DISCOUNTS FOR SSR TEACHERS AND VOLUME PURCHASES

ORDERS AND PAYMENT

Payment must be made by check or money order in U.S. funds. Please allow 2-3 weeks for delivery. Send your order including your name, address, phone number and e-mail address to:

Celestial Wellspring Publications	Phone:	800-966-5857 • 503-469-9292
6107 SW Murray Blvd., PMB213	Fax:	503-469-9393
Beaverton, Oregon 97008-4467	E-mail:	awakener@celestialwellspring.com

COMPANION MATERIALS

Other companion materials may become available soon, including:

- a video of Diane Ruth Shewmaker demonstrating the SSR attunements
- other SKHM Shenu items

For more information about these and other related products, please visit the website.

www.celestialwellspring.com